Contents

Preface and Acknowledgements

Preface

This small volume is not intended as a comprehensive textbook of respiratory medicine and physiology. Rather its purpose is to provide the relevant facts concerning respiratory problems that the senior student, house physician or registrar is likely to meet. The information is laid out clearly and economically to facilitate quick reference when on call in the small hours of the morning or when revising before examinations. The style is necessarily didactic to aid decision-making when faced with a sick patient who needs immediate diagnosis and treatment. The reader is therefore encouraged to use the blank sheets at the end of each chapter for personal notes and additions. The book is designed to be dipped into for reference rather than read cover to cover and to aid this a small amount of repetition has been introduced to enable each section to stand on its own.

Acknowledgements

I am very grateful to Mr R. Phillips and his staff in the Department of Medical Photography of the Middlesex Hospital Medical School for their work in producing the vast majority of the photographs and X-rays in this book. I would also like to thank Lydia Malim for drawing the illustrations, Mr Michael Newman for the microbiological photographs, Dr S. Wilson and Dr J. Adam for their help and advice concerning the choice of original X-rays. Dr J. Cotes has kindly given his permission to reproduce the nomograms of normal values. I thank Clement Clark Ltd for permission to reproduce normal values of peak flows and photographs of peak flow meters and gauges, and W.B. Pharmaceuticals for permission to use four endoscopic pictures. I am greatly endebted to Miss Michelle Brooks and Mrs Sue Chan for all their valiant work in typing the manuscript, and to Dr Anton Pozniak for his helpful criticism. Lastly I am grateful to Penny, my wife, for her help and advice throughout the numerous drafts of this book.

1.0 History

1.0 History

1.1 Introduction

A full careful history from a patient is essential; often the diagnosis can be made from this alone. It is very important to find out how incapacitated the patient is by his symptoms, and the extent to which the quality of his life is limited. Physical examination will confirm or refute the possibilities suggested by the clinical history, and simple investigations, particularly a chest X-ray, ECG and pulmonary function tests, will support the history and examination. In some cases, more refined tests such as lung biopsy, will be necessary in order to arrive at a definitive diagnosis.

It is a peculiarity of respiratory medicine, that often when the patient has been referred to the hospital physician because of an abnormal chest X-ray, the diagnosis may be self-evident even before the patient is seen. Nevertheless, a history is essential, even if only for the important reason to find out how the patient's disease is affecting his life and that of his family.

It is assumed that the readers of this book will have already developed their own method of taking a full history and performing a physical examination. Thus, the aim here is merely to highlight the respiratory implications of some of the findings.

1.2 The patient's background

Age

Certain diseases and conditions are more likely to occur at different times of life.

Younger patients (up to 30 years of age)
- atopic asthma
- pneumothorax
- congenital heart disease
- sarcoidosis
- cystic fibrosis

Older patients (over 50 years of age)
- intrinsic asthma

1.0 History

1.2 The patient's background

- ischaemic heart disease
- chronic bronchitis and emphysema
- pneumoconiosis
- cancer of the lung
- cryptogenic fibrosing alveolitis

Occupation

A full occupational history of past and present employment is essential. In particular, exposure to dust or chemicals should be noted. Occupations especially at risk are:
- coal miners
- farmers
- asbestos workers
- workers with epoxy resins or isocyanates

Racial origin

Immigrants, especially those of Asian extraction, appear to be especially at risk from tuberculosis, in particular during the first 2–3 years after arriving in the UK.

1.3 Presenting symptoms

It is important to obtain the full history of the present illness. Ascertain when the patient was last completely well, and whether he has had any similar illness in the past. The main triad of respiratory symptoms are shortness of breath, cough and chest pain. Enquire carefully about these, regardless of whether or not the patient volunteers their presence.

Breathlessness

Shortness of breath is one of the most common respiratory symptoms. It is subjective, being impossible to quantify. The feeling of breathlessness is probably related to an increase in the work of breathing; the neurological pathways which give rise to this feeling arise not within the lungs themselves, but in the muscles of the chest wall. It is important to stress that breathlessness and blood gas abnormalities or lung function tests bear little direct relationship to one another.

1.0 History

1.3 Presenting symptoms

Ascertain the severity of breathlessness
- is it true shortness of breath or merely a feeling of discomfort or pain in the chest?
- how severe is the breathlessness?
- how far can the patient walk before stopping?
- how many stairs can he climb?
- what effect does it have on the patient's job, social and sex life?
- is orthopnoea present? If so, how many pillows does the patient need?
- does the patient ever feel so breathless that he feels about to die?
- have there been any witnesses to the attacks? Did the patient look blue?

Causes
There are numerous causes of breathlessness. Respiratory or cardiac diseases account for the vast majority.

Common respiratory causes
The common respiratory causes are shown in Tables 1 and 2.

Left ventricular failure (LVF). This is the most common cardiac cause, being the result of one of the following:
- ischaemic heart disease
- valvular heart disease
- hypertension
- cardiomyopathies
- overtransfusion

Neuromuscular diseases. These are rare causes of breathlessness, but respiratory embarrassment must be remembered in each of the following:
- severe scoliosis
- ankylosing spondylitis
- poliomyelitis
- Guillain-Barré syndrome
- myasthenia gravis

Renal failure. This maybe a cause of hyperventilation due either to the central stimulus of acidosis, or pulmonary oedema caused by fluid retention or severe hypoalbuminaemia

1.3 Presenting symptoms

Table 1 Causes and features of breathlessness.

	Onset			Recurrent episodes common	Exposure or Occupation related	Nocturnal attacks
	Acute (hours)	Subacute (days or weeks)	Chronic (months/years)			
Pulmonary						
Asthma attack	+	+		+	+	+
Chronic bronchitis and emphysema			+	+	+	
Pneumonia	+	+				
TB		+				
Interstitial disease inc pneumoconiosis			+		+	
Pleural effusions		+		(+)		
Pneumothorax	+				+	
Lung cancer		+		+	+	
Allergic alveolitis	+			+	+	
Pulmonary embolism	+	+		(+)		
Bronchiectasis			+	+		

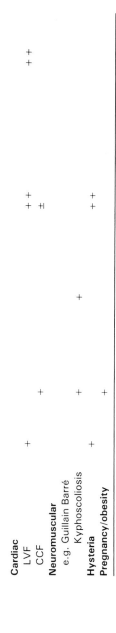

1.3 Presenting symptoms

Table 2 Associated features of breathlessness.

	Wheeze	Purulent sputum	Haemoptysis	Smoking related	Chest pain	Peripheral oedema
Pulmonary						
Asthma attack	+ +	±				
Chronic bronchitis and emphysema	+ +	+ +	±	+ +		Cor pulmonale
Pneumonia		+ +	+ +		+ +	
TB		+	+ +			
Interstitial disease inc pneumoconiosis						
Pleural effusions					+	
Pneumothorax					+ +	
Lung cancer			+ +	+ +	+ +	
Allergic alveolitis	±	±		+ +		
Pulmonary embolism			+ +	+	+	Deep vein thrombosis
Bronchiectasis	+	+ +	+ +			
Cardiac						
LVF	+		±	+ +	±	
CCF				+ +	±	+ +
Neuromuscular e.g. Guillain Barré						
Kyphoscoliosis						
Hysteria						
Pregnancy/obesity						

1.3 Presenting symptoms

Diabetes mellitus. This can cause:
- hyperventilation (air hunger) due to central stimulation with severe ketoacidosis

Anaemia or altitude. These factors may cause breathlessness due to:
- reduced oxygen-carrying capacity of blood in anaemia and due to the reduced ambient P_{IO_2} at high altitude
- acute pulmonary oedema (mountain sickness) at very high altitude (over 17 000 ft), especially in those who are not acclimatized

Timing
- severe asthma and left ventricular failure are more frequent at night, particularly in the early hours of the morning
- occupational asthma is worse during the week when exposed to the antigen and better at weekends when at home
- bronchitis is worse in winter; atopic asthma is worse in spring and summer in those allergic to pollens; perennial in those allergic to house dust mite and autumnal in allergic aspergillosis

Alleviating or aggravating factors
The doctor should ask whether exercise, allergens, excitement, cold air, hyperventilation, sexual intercourse or coughing aggravate symptoms. Do β agonist aerosols or any other therapies alleviate symptoms? Do any drugs make things worse, e.g. aspirin or β blockers?

Causes of wheeze

Wheeze is the noisy musical sound caused by turbulent airflow through narrowed bronchi and bronchioles. As these tend to be shorter and narrower in expiration, that is when wheezing is more pronounced.

Wheezing occurs in conditions associated with airways obstruction. The following causes are common:
- asthma (at any age)
- chronic bronchitis and emphysema (smokers over 50)
- bronchiolitis (children)

(Occasionally wheeze is caused by left ventricular failure —
'cardiac asthma')

The airways obstruction is produced by a mixture of bronchial
smooth muscle spasm, oedema and mucus production. In any
patient who has a wheeze, elicit the following points:
- is the wheeze persistent (chronic bronchitis and emphysema)
  or intermittent (asthma)?
- nocturnal or on waking (asthma or LVF)?
- worse on exercise or hyperventilation (asthma)?
- related to dust or other allergens (asthma)?
- related to industrial exposure or di-isocyanates (asthma)?
- worse with drugs such as alcohol, aspirin, or β blockers
  (asthma)? β blockers may also precipitate LVF.

Wheeze is often associated with shortness of breath, and a
central non-anginal chest tightness. It is important to realize
that with very severe airways obstruction there can be so little
air moving in or out of the chest that turbulent flow does not
occur, and hence there is no wheeze. This is the 'quiet' or
'silent' chest.

Causes of stridor

Stridor is the term applied to noisy respiration which is always
worse during inspiration — this is caused by central large
airways obstruction. Common causes are as follows:
- carcinoma of the larynx, trachea, or major bronchus
- tracheal stenosis, post-tracheostomy, or from extrinsic
  compression, i.e. goitre
- laryngeal oedema, i.e. angio-oedema

Stridor can be accentuated by asking the patient first to cough,
then to inspire through an open mouth.

Cough

- try to find out whether this arises in the chest or whether it
  arises in the oro- or naso pharynx (or even due to external
  ear disease stimulating the vagus nerve!)
- how long has it been present? Extensive investigation is not

warranted for coughs in the first 2 weeks, only if they persist
- when does it occur? — day or night, or both. Most coughs are worse at night or first thing on waking
- is it persistent or intermittent?
- is the cough painful?
- is there any possibility of foreign body inhalation?

Causes
The following are diseases which often present with cough:

Acute cough. If there is a history of less than two weeks, acute cough may be caused by:
- tracheitis, viral or bacterial
- bronchitis, viral or bacterial
- bronchiolitis, viral or bacterial
- pneumonia, viral or bacterial
- asthma
- pulmonary oedema
- pulmonary embolism
- whooping cough
- foreign body inhalation
- onset of chronic cough

Chronic cough. Causes of chronic cough include:
- chronic bronchitis
- asthma
- carcinoma
- tuberculosis
- interstitial (acinar) lung disease
- bronchiectasis
- foreign body inhalation
- benign tumour
- whooping cough
- mediastinal lesions, e.g. nodes, aneurysms
- habit cough

Haemoptysis

Virtually all patients who consult their doctors about haemoptysis are worried about the possibility of lung cancer, though fortunately only about 3% of cases will, in fact, be suffering from this. Nevertheless, haemoptysis is a symptom which should be specifically asked about in all patients, and which, when detected, always requires careful investigation. It is important to differentiate haemoptysis from haematemesis or nose bleeding. Was the blood definitely coughed up or was it vomited? Was it merely from the nasopharynx? Was there any bleeding from the nose?

Despite investigation, haemoptysis remains unexplained in over 40% of patients. However, the following causes must first be excluded.

Causes

Common pulmonary causes of haemoptysis are (see also Table 3):
- acute tracheobronchitis
- pneumonia
- lung cancer
- tuberculosis
- pulmonary infarction
- bronchiectasis

Rarer pulmonary causes of haemoptysis may be:
- abscess
- aspergilloma
- apical fibrosis
- foreign bodies
- benign tumours
- hereditary haemorrhagic telangiectasia

Non pulmonary causes
- left ventricular failure
- mitral stenosis
- blood dyscrasias

Chest pain

Causes
Chest pain is a very common medical symptom. Several different types of pain occur. The character of the pain usually gives a clue to the cause.

Angina pectoris. Caused by ischaemic heart disease, this is worse on exertion. It is a squeezing pain, often radiating to the neck and left arm, which is relieved by rest.

1.3 Presenting symptoms

Table 3 Clinical features of common causes of haemoptysis.

	Purulent sputum	Repetitive specks or streaks of blood	Pleuritic pain	Possible cause of massive haemoptysis	Recurrent over several years
Acute tracheobronchitis	+				
Pneumonia	+		+		
Lung cancer		+		+	
Tuberculosis	+			+	
Pulmonary infarct			+		
Bronchiectasis	+	+		+	+

1.3   Presenting symptoms

Pleurisy.   The pain is aggravated by respiration. It is often very severe and described as knifelike. A pleural rub may be present. Involvement of the diaphragmatic pleura causes pain to be referred to the shoulder tip. Pleural pain is caused by:
• pneumonia
• pulmonary infarction
• pneumothorax
• cancer
• rib fractures

Retrosternal pain.   There is often a burning discomfort in acute tracheitis. Oesophagitis or hiatus hernia are aggravated by eating and may be related to posture. A dull pain may be caused by mediastinal lesions such as lymphadenopathy from a cancer or lymphoma.

Pain in intercostal nerve distribution may be caused by:
• thoracic vertebral collapse — local tenderness over dorsal spine
• *Herpes zoster* (shingles) — typical rash
• Bornholm disease (coxsackie B) — tender intercostal muscles
• costochondritis

Pericarditis.   Central poorly localized tightness related to posture and movement. A pericardial rub is often present and the patient may be febrile.

1.4   Important coexisting symptoms

Although breathlessness, cough and chest pain are the most common presenting symptoms of respiratory disease, other important symptoms often coexist with these.

Fever

Common respiratory causes are:
• acute infections — bronchitis or pneumonia
• chronic infections such as tuberculosis
• lung cancer or lymphoma

1.0 History

1.4 Important coexisting symptoms

Poor appetite and weight loss

These are very important symptoms which warrant further investigation. Common lung diseases associated with weight loss are:
• emphysema
• lung cancer
• chronic infection such as TB

Ankle swelling

This may be caused by:
• cardiac failure — congestive cardiac failure or cor pulmonale
• renal failure
• hepatic failure
• hypoalbuminaemia — nutritional
• carbon dioxide retention due to chronic obstructive bronchitis
• lymphoedema

Deep vein thrombosis

Characterized by painful swelling of one leg (iliac thrombosis may cause bilateral leg oedema).

Palpitations

These may signify:
• cardiac disease
• thyrotoxicosis
• anxiety state
• phaeochromocytoma
• drug overdose — e.g. β agonists

1.5 A full systematic enquiry

The previous sections cover the respiratory and cardiovascular systems but it is important to make the usual enquiries about the other systems — alimentary, genitourinary, central nervous and locomotor systems.

1.6   Past medical history

- ask for details of all previous illnesses and operations or radiotherapy together with details of any hospitalization
- has the patient ever had a chest X-ray? Why? When? Where? — a previous X-ray may save a lot of excess investigation
- has the patient ever been medically examined for a job, the armed services or life insurance? Were any abnormalities such as heart murmurs or hypertension found?
- ask after childhood illnesses — particularly rheumatic fever, measles and whooping cough
- has the patient ever had hay fever, urticaria, eczema or asthma?
- is he diabetic, has he ever had anaemia or thyroid disease?
- has he ever had any heart or lung disease?
- has there been any chest surgery? Why?
- has he ever had tuberculosis of any organ? When? Where was it treated? For how long? With drugs? With surgery? (full details are essential)
- if there has been any surgery in the past, try to ascertain by careful questioning whether this was for a benign or malignant condition — often the answer will mean that contact needs to be made with previous medical attendants

1.7   Family history

Is there any other chest disease in the family? What type?
- tuberculosis — may spread with close contact
- asthma — hereditary (ask also after hay fever and eczema)
- emphysema — hereditary if due to α_1 antitrypsin deficiency
- cystic fibrosis? — hereditary

Other diseases which may run in families include hypertension, diabetes mellitus, thyroid disease and ankylosing spondylitis.

Record age and state of health of near relatives or the cause of death of any who have died.

1.8 Social history

- how much does the patient smoke? Record past and present consumption (1 pack year = 20 cigarettes per day for a year)
- how much alcohol is consumed?
- record country of origin. How long in UK?
- what type of accommodation does he live in?
- how many stairs are there? Is there a lift?
- married or single? Number of children and their ages?
- are there any pets? — many, such as cats and dogs, might aggravate asthma; others such as pigeons or budgerigars may cause pulmonary fibrosis in some people. Parrots can be a vector for ornithoses
- does he have any hobbies?
- any recent travel or contact with infectious diseases?
- in some patients it is necessary to ask delicately about family, financial and sexual problems

1.9 Current medications

All medications should be documented, including oral contraceptives. How long has the patient been taking any current medication (especially steroid therapy)? Ask what previous medications have been used in order to avoid prescribing drugs which have been found to be ineffective.

1.10 Allergies

All known allergens, including drugs, must be recorded. Ask the patient directly whether he is allergic to drugs such as antibiotics. Record allergies in capitals on the front of the notes and on the patient's treatment chart.

2.0 Physical examination

2.0 Physical examination

2.1 General appearance

2.1 General appearance

Before the patient is seen in out-patients or in a hospital ward it is essential that his physician should have to hand information concerning his body temperature, body weight, blood pressure, pulse and respiratory rates and routine urine analysis.

While the history is being taken the patient should be carefully observed to note the following points:
- does the patient look ill?
- is he in pain?
- level of consciousness or presence of confusion
- is the patient breathless?
- the character of breathing and the presence of audible wheezing or stridor
- cyanosis — best seen in the tongue
- signs of overt weight loss
- the use of accessory muscles of respiration
- the presence of pallor, anaemia or polycythaemia

If breathlessness is the main symptom, but the patient does not appear breathless during examination, try exercising the patient whilst walking alongside him. Note whether the symptom occurs and whether there is any sign of cyanosis.

On full examination the following signs should be noted with particular reference to respiratory symptoms.

2.2 Cyanosis

Central cyanosis

Best seen as blue discolouration of the tongue, cyanosis implies arterial hypoxaemia. Cyanosis is first seen when arterial saturation falls to 85% (Pa_{O_2} < 50–60 mmHg, 7–8 kPa). Chronic hypoxia is a potent stimulus for erythropoietin secretion thus leading to secondary polycythaemia and accentuation of the cyanosis. Over 5 g/dl of reduced haemoglobin must be present before cyanosis is recognizable; thus it is more difficult to recognize with anaemia, and easier to recognize with polycythaemia. Some other pigments cause a

2.0 Physical examination

2.2 Cyanosis

---

bluish appearance which may be mistaken for cyanosis, notably sulph- or met-haemoglobinaemia caused by drugs such as phenacetin, sulphonamides or primaquine.

Causes
The common causes of central cyanosis are:
- chronic bronchitis and emphysema
- pulmonary embolism
- left ventricular failure
- right to left congenital cardiac shunts

Peripheral cyanosis

This is recognizable by blue fingers and toes but with a normal pink tongue and is found in:
- normal people in cold weather
- Raynauds syndrome
- peripheral vascular disease

2.3 Finger clubbing

Although the reason is unknown, there are numerous conditions which lead to the fingers acquiring this characteristic shape (Figs 1 and 2). The early stages of clubbing are very difficult to differentiate from normal appearances, whereas the advanced stages are very obvious. The features to look for are:
- loss of nailbed angle
- increase in the size of the distal phalanx
- fluctuant nailbed
- increased nail curvature

Causes

Neoplastic
- bronchial carcinoma
- mesothelioma

Infective
- bronchiectasis, including cystic fibrosis
- lung abscess
- empyema

2.0 Physical examination

2.3 Finger clubbing

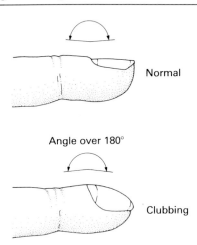

Normal

Angle over 180°

Clubbing

Fig. 1 *Finger clubbing. Note the increase in the nailbed angle as well as the increased curvature of the nail and swelling of the terminal part of the digit.*

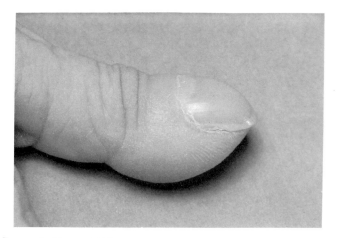

Fig. 2 *Finger clubbing.*

2.0   Physical examination

2.3   Finger clubbing

- chronic pulmonary tuberculosis
- subacute bacterial endocarditis

Fibrotic
- asbestosis
- cryptogenic fibrosing alveolitis

Cyanotic congenital heart disease
- any with right-to-left shunt

Gastrointestinal
- primary biliary cirrhosis
- Crohn's disease
- ulcerative colitis

Congenital (autosomal dominant)

Hypertrophic pulmonary osteoarthropathy

This is a rare condition associated with clubbing. The characteristics are those of pain and swelling of the wrists and ankles with subperiosteal new bone formation seen on X-ray examination. It is most commonly associated with bronchial carcinoma.

2.4   Extremities

Hands and wrists

- warm hands and tachycardia (causes: fever, hypoxia, hypercapnia, cardiac failure, thyrotoxicosis or anxiety)
- fine tremor — β agonist therapy or anxiety
- flapping tremor (CO_2 retention or liver failure)

Head and neck

Look for:
- fundi — check for papilloedema (hypercapnia or raised intracranial pressure)
- Horner's syndrome (Fig. 3) (ptosis, loss of sweating, constricted pupil — can be caused by an apical carcinoma

invading the sympathetic plexus)
- character and volume of carotid pulse — particularly important in aortic valve disease
- raised JVP — pulsatile: right heart failure
  — non-pulsatile: superior vena cava obstruction
- tracheal position
- distance from thyroid cartilage to suprasternal notch (reduced with chronic airways obstruction)
- goitres
- cervical and supraclavicular fossa lymph nodes — local sepsis, glandular fever, tuberculosis, sarcoidosis, lymphoma, other malignancies
- phrenic crush scars
- tuberculous node excision scars

2.5   Chest inspection (Fig. 4)

Skin

Look for any scars, rashes, dilated veins, skin nodules, subcutaneous nodules or vasculitis.

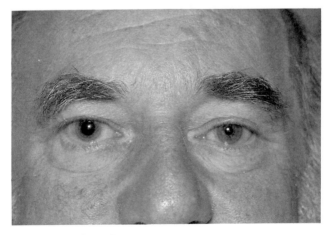

Fig. 3 *Horner's syndrome.*

2.0   Physical examination

2.5   Chest inspection

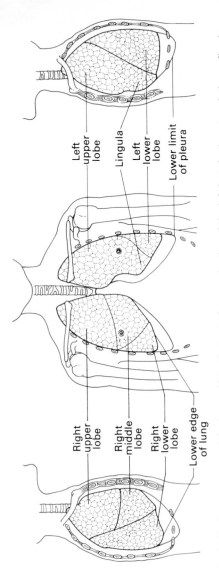

Fig. 4 Surface anatomy of the lungs. Note that anterior examination of the left lung is almost entirely confined to the upper lobe, and on the right to the upper and middle lobes, the latter being situated just under the right nipple in the male. On the back examination is mainly of the lower lobes which also stretch round into the axillae.

2.0 Physical examination

2.5 Chest inspection

Shape

Look for indications of the following:
- pigeon (pectus carinatum) or funnel chest (pectus excavatum). Neither of these usually causes any problems
- barrel chest (increased AP diameter together with use of accessory muscles) (Fig. 5). Found in diseases associated with airways obstruction, such as chronic bronchitis and emphysema and chronic inadequately treated asthma
- any evidence of previous chest surgery or injury
- flattening over areas of local fibrosis or collapse or with excision of upper lobes
- kyphoscoliosis. Scoliosis causes more problems than kyphosis due to V/Q mismatch which leads to pulmonary hypertension

Movement

- decreased unilaterally on the same side as any focal abnormality
- poor bilateral chest movement (less than 5 cm expansion can occur with severe airways obstruction or diseases such as ankylosing spondylitis)
- prolonged expiration together with rib indrawing in inspiration; both suggest airways obstruction

2.6 Palpation (Fig. 6)

Check for the position of the trachea. This is pulled towards areas of fibrosis or collapse and pushed away from large pleural effusions or a tension pneumothorax.

2.7 Percussion (Fig. 6)

Reduced resonance

This occurs over any area of increased density:
- pleural effusion (stony dullness)
- pleural thickening or tumour
- pneumonia (consolidation)

Table 4 Physical signs in chest disease.

	Inspection and palpation			Percussion	Breath sounds	Auscultation	
	Shape of chest	Movement	Position of trachea			Character of breath sounds	Additional sounds
Airways obstruction, e.g. asthma or bronchitis	Hyperinflated ↑ AP diameter	Bilaterally decreased	Central	Resonant	Decreased	Normal	Rhonchi (wheezes) mainly expiratory
Lobar collapse, e.g. foreign body or carcinoma	Normal	Decreased on side affected	Towards collapse	Dull	Decreased or absent	—	—
Lobar consolidation, e.g. pneumonia	Normal	Decreased on side affected	Central	Dull	Increased	Bronchial	Crepitations (crackles) ocassionally pleural rub
Pneumothorax	Normal	Decreased on side affected	Central or away from side if tension present	Hyper-resonant	Decreased	Normal	Occasional pneumothorax click if left-sided
Pleural effusion	Normal	Decreased on side affected	Away from effusion	Stony dull	Decreased or absent	Occasionally bronchial above level of effusion	Occasionally pleural rub
Localized fibrosis	Flattening of side affected	Decreased on side affected	Towards fibrosis	Dull	Increased only if upper lobe	Bronchial	Crepitations (crackles)
Diffuse interstitial	Normal	Diminished bilaterally	Central	Resonant	Normal	Normal	Crepitations (crackles)

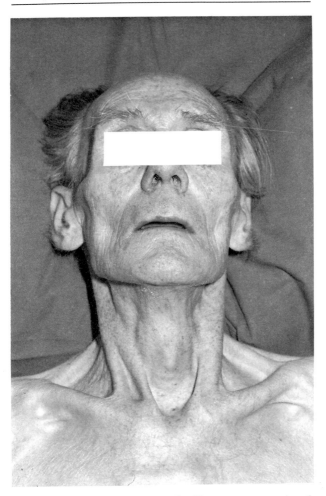

Fig. 5 *Patient with emphysema using his accessory muscles of respiration.*

2.0 Physical examination

2.7 Percussion

- local fibrosis
- large lung tumours

Increased resonance

Increased resonance is due to relative increase of air in the chest:
- airways obstruction with gas trapping, e.g. emphysema
- a pneumothorax

2.8 Auscultation (Fig. 6)

Breath sounds

Diminished breath sounds
Diminished breath sounds are found either because of poor ventilation:
- airways obstruction — bronchitis, emphysema and asthma
- respiratory depression by drugs (i.e. opiates, barbiturates)

or because of increased separation of the stethoscope from the bronchial tree:
- obese patients
- pleural effusion or tumour
- bronchial tumour
- pneumothorax
- lobar collapse

Increased and altered character (bronchial breathing)
- over consolidated lung (pneumonia)
- at the top level of a pleural effusion
- over dense localized fibrosis
- lung abscess with a patent bronchus

Extra sounds

Wheezes (rhonchi)
These usually occur in expiration and imply airways narrowing:
- asthma
- chronic bronchitis and emphysema

2.8 Auscultation

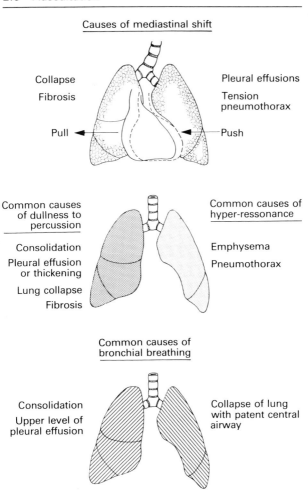

Causes of mediastinal shift

Collapse
Fibrosis

Pleural effusions

Tension
pneumothorax

Pull ◄— —Push

Common causes
of dullness to
percussion

Consolidation

Pleural effusion
or thickening

Lung collapse

Fibrosis

Common causes of
hyper-ressonance

Emphysema

Pneumothorax

Common causes of
bronchial breathing

Consolidation

Upper level of
pleural effusion

Collapse of lung
with patent central
airway

Fig. 6 *Common causes of abnormal physical signs in the chest.*

2.8 Auscultation

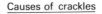

Causes of crackles

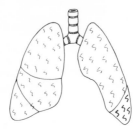

Fine		Medium
Pneumonia		Fibrosis
Pulmonary oedema		Bronchiectasis sometimes
Bronchiolitis		Coarse
Tuberculosis		Bronchiectasis

Causes of wheezes

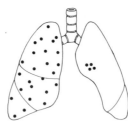

Generalised

Airways obstruction

Chronic bronchitis or asthma

Localised

Mucus (clears on coughing)

Local narrowing

e.g. Neoplasms, inflammation, lymph glands, foreign body

Fig. 6 *Common causes of abnormal physical signs in the chest.*

- bronchiolitis
- left ventricular failure (occasionally)
- tumours and foreign bodies

Tumours and foreign bodies should particularly be considered if there is a localized fixed monophonic wheeze which is not abolished by coughing.

Fine crackles (crepitations) — inspiratory
These signify any of three causes:
- pulmonary oedema (left heart failure)
- early or localized pneumonia
- fibrosing alveolitis

Medium or coarse crackles (râles) — inspiratory
These are found in:
- bronchiectasis
- severe pulmonary oedema

2.8 Auscultation

Pleural friction rub
This is found with pleural involvement by infection, infarction or tumour.

2.9 Sputum

In any patient with suspected respiratory disease, enquire about the production of sputum.

Direct inspection of the sputum is essential. A few of the typical appearances include:
• white mucoid sputum in chronic bronchitis or asthma
• purulent green or yellow sputum may imply viral or bacterial infection (NB eosinophils may also give a yellow-green appearance in asthma without infection)
• the presence of blood (haemoptysis) should be looked for carefully
• frothy white or pink sputum suggests pulmonary oedema

2.10 Cardiovascular system

As respiratory symptoms are often caused by cardiovascular disease a full, careful examination of the heart and cardiovascular system is essential (for a full account see Swanton R.H. (1984) *Pocket Consultant on Cardiology*. Blackwell Scientific Publications, Oxford). A brief checklist of the main points to watch out for follows.

Left ventricular failure

• tachycardia (unless in heart block or when taking β blockers)
• enlarged heart
• gallop rhythm (III or IV heart sound)
• basal crepitations (crackles)
• pulsus alternans

Common causes
• ischaemic heart disease — angina, abnormal ECG
• valvular heart disease — characteristic murmurs
• hypertension — check BP and fundi, loud A_2
• fluid overload due to overtransfusion, or renal failure

2.0 Physical examination

2.10 Cardiovascular system

- anaemia
- thyrotoxicosis

Right ventricular failure

- elevated jugular venous pressure
- peripheral oedema
- enlarged right ventricle
- often loud P_2
- hepatomegaly

Common causes
- congestive cardiac failure (secondary to left heart failure) due to the causes listed above
- cor pulmonale because of pulmonary hypertension caused by chronic lung disease, e.g. chronic bronchitis, massive or repeated pulmonary embolism, severe kyphoscoliosis, and in the late stages of emphysema and pulmonary fibrosis

Peripheral oedema without right ventricular failure may occur in chronic bronchitis due to CO_2 retention.

2.11 Other systems

A complete examination of the other systems is essential, a few examples related to respiratory disease are given.

Abdomen (including rectal examination)

Hepatomegaly
- right heart failure
- liver metastases
- lymphoma
- sarcoidosis (or TB)

Splenomegaly
- sarcoidosis
- tuberculosis
- lymphoma
- endocarditis
- chronic liver disease

2.0 Physical examination

2.11 Other systems

Gastrointestinal tract
- cancers may metastasize to the lungs

Genitourinary

Renal failure may present as pulmonary oedema due to Na^+ and water retention.

Renal and genital tumours often metastasize to the lungs.

Locomotor

Rheumatoid arthritis, SLE and PAN commonly affect the lung and pleura. Bone pain due to secondaries is common in lung cancer. Arthralgia may occur with sarcoidosis.

Central nervous system

Severe hypoxia and hypercapnia may cause drowsiness, confusion and even coma. Papilloedema and flapping tremor can also be caused. Lung cancer may present due to cerebral secondaries (epilepsy or focal signs) or through non-metastatic cerebral and cerebellar degeneration. Peripheral neuropathies may be found with connective tissue disorders and rarely with sarcoidosis and lung cancer. Sarcoidosis is a common cause of a Bell's palsy (LMN VII cranial nerve).

Skin

Erythema nodosum	— sarcoidosis
	— tuberculosis (rare)
Lupus pernio	— sarcoidosis
Lupus vulgaris	— tuberculosis
Lupus erythematosus	— SLE
Bazin's disease	— tuberculosis
Nodules	— rheumatoid arthritis
	— skin secondaries from lung cancer
Vasculitis	— scleroderma
	— SLE
Plaques	— sarcoidosis
Sclerodactyly, Telangiectasia and Raynauds	— scleroderma

3.0 Investigations

3.0 Investigations

3.1 Sputum

3.1 Sputum

Mucus is continuously produced throughout the bronchial tree. It lines the respiratory tract, providing a protective coating onto which inhaled foreign particles deposit. The particles are carried up by ciliary action towards the mouth. In normal subjects, this colourless mucus is swallowed. When there is an increase in mucus secretion, either because of bronchial infection or irritation, the patient becomes aware of sputum production which he then expectorates. Excessive sputum production is abnormal, and needs investigation. The starting point is the examination of the sputum itself.

Collection

To obtain the maximum diagnostic information from sputum, it is important to collect a good sample in the first place. It is strongly recommended that the doctor either collects the sample himself, or gets a trained physiotherapist to collect it following therapy.

Appearance

Clear, sticky mucoid sputum of variable volume is typical of chronic bronchitis with no infection. Thick, green or yellow non-sticky sputum is found with pulmonary infection, e.g. pneumonia, abscess or bronchiectasis. There is usually copious production. With infective episodes of bronchitis sputum may be mucopurulent or frankly purulent. Eosinophilia in asthma may also impart a yellow colour without infection. Black sputum occurs with coal mining, smoke inhalation or very heavy cigarette smoking. Copious frothy white or pink sputum is characteristic of pulmonary oedema. Haemoptysis should also be noted and investigated. 'Rusty' sputum is typically caused by a pneumococcal pneumonia. Bronchial casts (Curschmann's spirals) are sometimes expectorated in asthma. Mucus plugs and casts are found in bronchopulmonary aspergillosis.

Microscopy

Gram stain
Note cell constituents, e.g. polymorphs in infection and eosinophils in asthma.

3.0 Investigations

3.1 Sputum

Common bacterial pathogens. The following common bacterial pathogens may be found after Gram stain:

- *Streptococcus pneumonia*
  (Pneumococcus) ⎫
- *Staphylococcus aureus* ⎬ Gram-positive cocci
- *Haemophilus influenzae* ⎫
- *Klebsiella pneumonia* ⎬ Gram-negative rods

Rarely found pathogens. These include:
- fungal hyphae, e.g. *Aspergillus fumigatus*

Ziehl-Neelsen and Auramine stains
- mycobacterium tuberculosis

Cytology for neoplastic cells

Three sputum specimens should be examined for neoplastic cells. In good laboratories, 70% or more of lung cancers are diagnosable in this way. Post-bronchoscopy sputum collection has the highest yield. Asbestos bodies may be noted in those exposed (Fig. 7).

Absence of sputum

If patients with pneumonia or suspected TB are producing no sputum, it can be very helpful to obtain bronchial suckings and lavage via the fibreoptic bronchoscope and process them as one would sputum samples. In tuberculosis these methods have largely replaced laryngeal swabbings and gastric washings. Any washings should be done with sterile 0.9% saline, and not with tap water, because in some areas this contains non-pathogenic mycobacteria which may lead to diagnostic confusion.

3.2 Radiology

Plain chest X-ray (Figs 8 and 9)

It is essential for the physician to be able to interpret chest X-rays accurately. There are frequently abnormalities on a chest X-ray with no abnormal physical signs. The chest X-ray is the

3.0 Investigations

3.2 Radiology

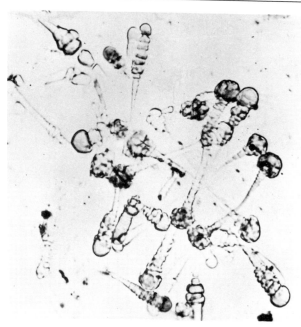

Fig. 7 *Asbestos bodies in the sputum of a patient with previous heavy asbestos exposure.*

most sensitive part of routine chest examination, except in cases of airways obstruction. Indeed, an abnormal X-ray is often the reason for the patient's initial referral to the hospital physician.

Departmental films are taken with the patient standing with the front of his chest against the X-ray cannister, the X-ray source being 2 m behind him (PA film). The film is taken in full inspiration. Emergency films are taken the other way round, with the X-ray source much closer to the patient (AP film). (It is important to realize that the heart size is magnified in AP film.) To interpret films accurately, it is best to develop a routine to read the films, checking them for the following:
• straightness
• penetration

3.2 Radiology

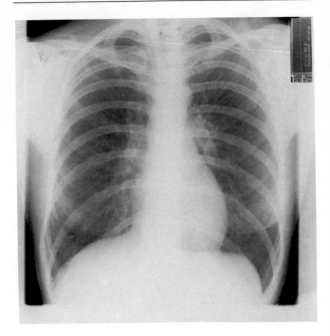

Fig. 8 *(a) Normal chest X-ray. Postero-anterior (PA)*

- adequate inspiration
- tracheal position
- shape and size of mediastinum and hilar shadows
- shape and size of heart
- position and shape of the diaphragm (check no air is immediately under it)
- lung fields, e.g. check position of fissures; check for infiltration; localized or generalized — look for mass lesions
- pleural abnormalities
- bone abnormalities
- soft tissue abnormalities
- see also checklist on page 70

Whenever a localized abnormality is seen, the relevant plain lateral (and possibly oblique) view is taken to localize the

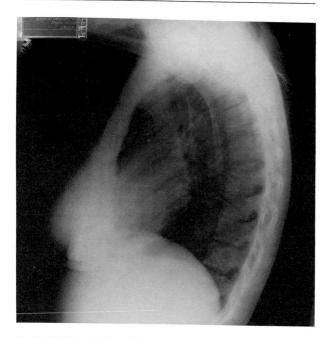

Fig. 8 *(b) Normal chest X-ray. Lateral.*

lesion. The following abnormalities are often seen on chest X-ray.

Consolidation
The consolidated lobe or segment is uniformly radiopaque. The borders coincide with the anatomical distribution although some degree of collapse is often present. In lingular or middle lobe consolidation the relevant heart border becomes indistinct.

Collapse
When a lobe collapses, the trachea and mediastinum are shifted towards the side of the collapse. Lobes collapse down into very small volumes and are uniformly radiopaque with characteristic patterns on the PA film. Although these shadows can be missed on a PA film alone they are usually obvious if a lateral is also available. Particular care must be taken not to

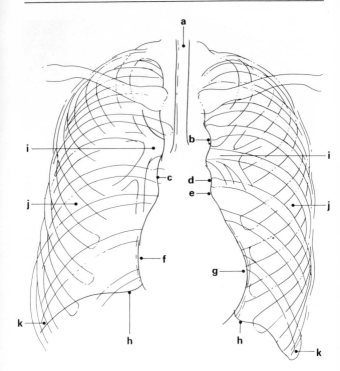

Fig. 9 *(a) Diagram of a normal chest X-ray. **a** trachea; **b** aortic arch; **c** superior vena cava; **d** pulmonary artery; **e** left atrial appendage; **f** right atrium; **g** left ventricle; **h** diaphragms — right 2 cm higher than the left; **i** hilar shadows consisting of pulmonary arteries and veins and lymph nodes; **j** lung fields; **k** costophrenic angles*

miss a left lower lobe collapse, it appears as a triangular shadow behind the heart on the lateral film, and on the PA film it causes a 'double' left heart border as it collapses behind the heart. Right middle lobe collapse may appear merely as a blurred right heart border on the PA film.

3.2   Radiology

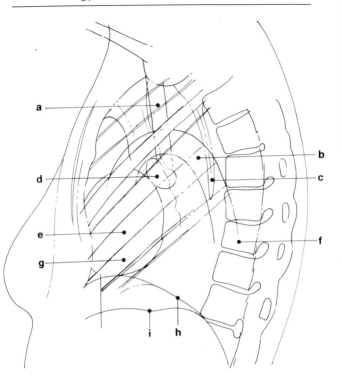

Fig. 9 *(b) Diagram of a lateral chest X-ray.* a *trachea;* b *aortic arch;* c *scapula;* d *hilum;* e *heart;* f *vertebral column;* g *rib;* h *right diaphragm;* i *left diaphragm*

Figures 11–27 illustrate various forms of consolidation and collapse.

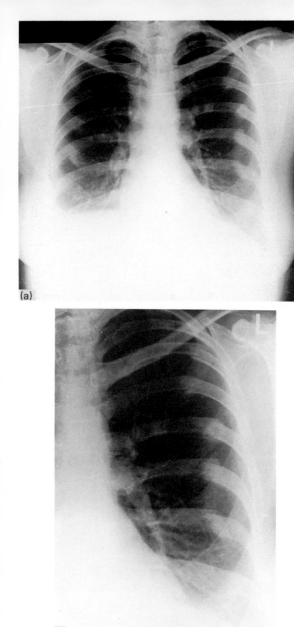

Fig. 10 *(a) Multiple left-side rib fractures following a car crash. (b) Close-up view of ribs.*

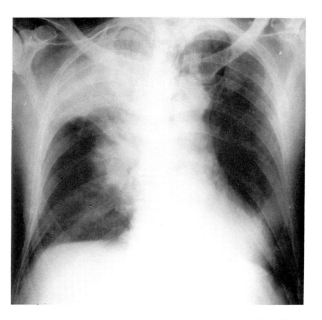

Fig. 11 *Right hilar mass with consolidation and partial collapse of the right upper lobe. Note the horizontal fissure is slightly elevated.*

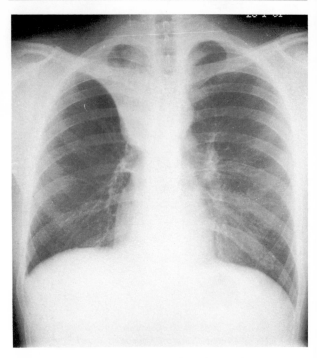

Fig. 12 *Right upper lobe collapse. Note the considerable elevation of the right hilum and spreading of the right lower zone lung vessels.*

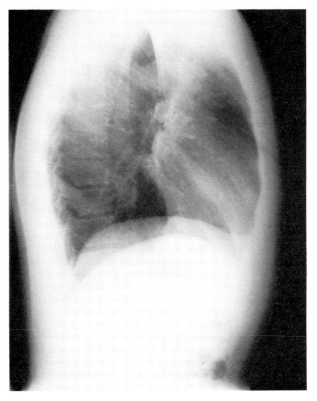

Fig. 13 *Right upper lobe collapse lateral view. Note the forward displacement of the oblique fissure and the elevation of the horizontal fissure.*

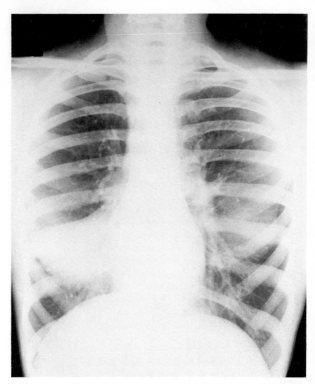

Fig. 14 *Right middle lobe collapse/consolidation. Note depression of the horizontal fissure and loss of definition of the right heart border.*

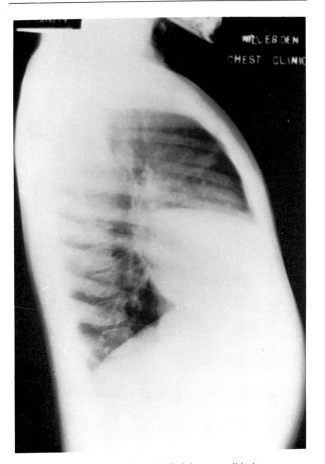

Fig. 15 *Lateral view — right middle lobe consolidation.*

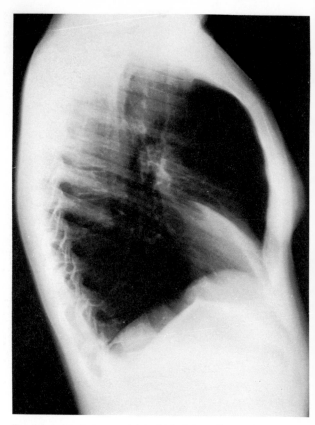

Fig. 16 *Lateral view — right middle lobe collapse. Note the very small volume the lobe now occupies.*

3.2 Radiology

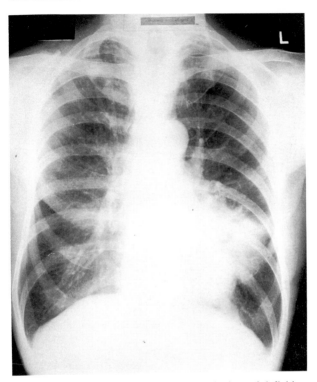

Fig. 17 *Consolidation of the lingula. Note the loss of definition of the left heart border.*

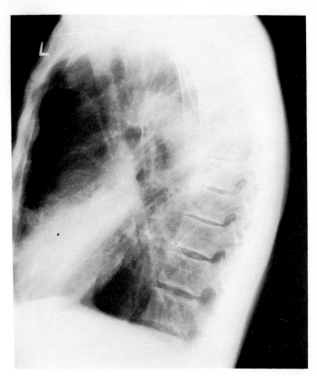

Fig. 18 *Lateral view — consolidation of the lingula.*

3.2 Radiology

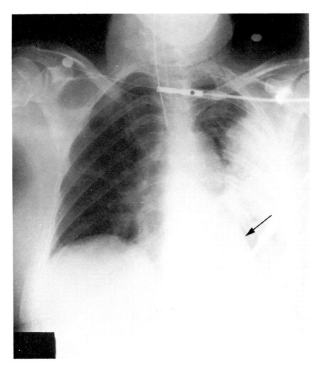

Fig. 19 *Left lower lobe consolidation. Note that the left heart border can still be defined (arrowed), note also the endotracheal tube and ECG leads.*

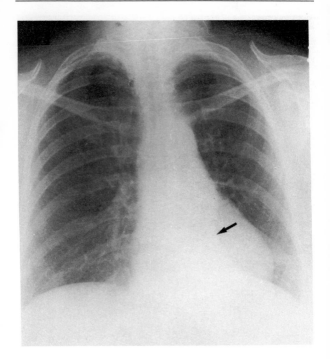

Fig. 20 *Left lower lobe collapse. Note the dense shadow seen through the heart.*

3.0 Investigations

3.2 Radiology

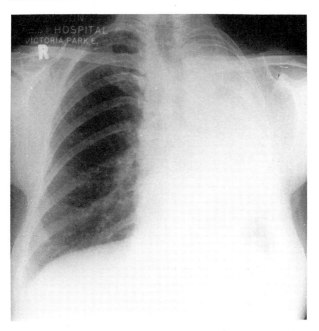

Fig. 21 *Complete collapse of the left lung due to a mucus plug in the main bronchus. Note the shift of the mediastinum and elevation of the left hemidiaphragm (and gastric air bubble) as well as opacification of the hemithorax.*

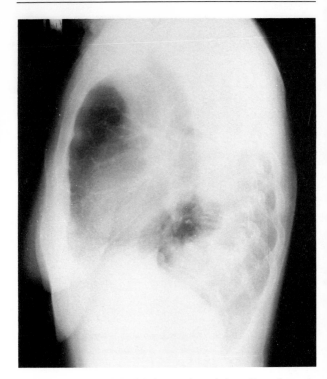

Fig. 22 *Collapse of the left lung — lateral view. Note that only the right hemidiaphragm is visualized.*

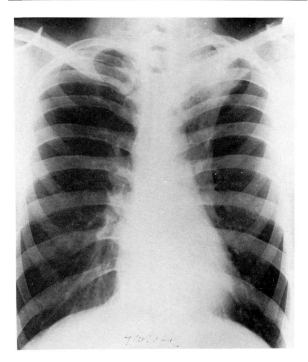

Fig. 23 *Left upper lobe consolidation with partial collapse.*

3.2 Radiology

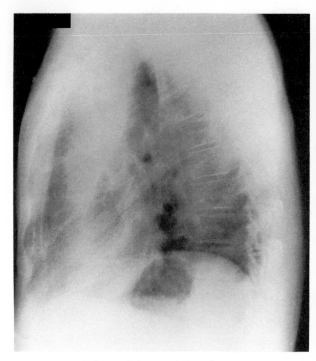

Fig. 24 *Lateral view — left upper lobe collapse.*

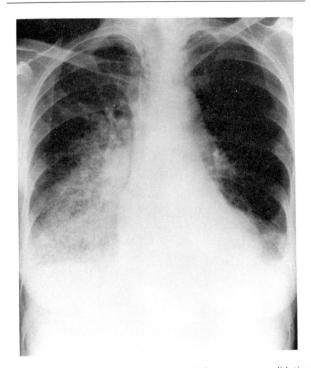

Fig. 25 *Right lower lobe consolidation (also some consolidation on the left).*

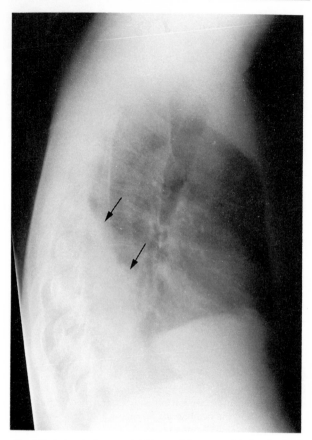

Fig. 26 *Lateral view — right lower lobe consolidation (partial). Note posterior radiodensity.*

3.2 Radiology

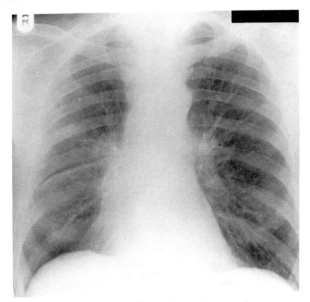

Fig. 27 *Right lower lobe collapse. Note downward displacement of the horizontal fissure.*

Pleural effusion (Figs 28 and 29)
About 300 ml of fluid is needed even to cause blunting of the costophrenic angles. Larger effusions show characteristic shadows with levels that rise in the axilla. Very large effusions may 'white out' the hemithorax. If there is any doubt as to whether the shadow is due to fluid, a lateral decubitus film can be taken to see if the level alters with gravity.

Pneumothorax
A distinct lung edge can be seen beyond which there are no lung markings. A small pneumothorax may only be obvious at the apex. Pneumothoraces *appear* larger on an expiratory film

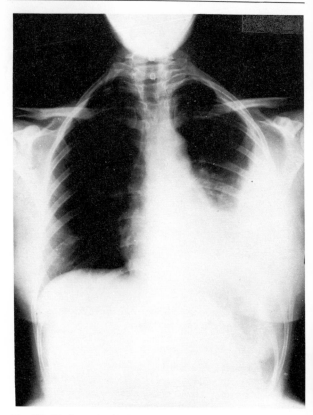

Fig. 28 *Medium-sized left pleural effusion. Note the curving upper border in the axilla.*

(when the intrapleural pressure is highest) because the intrapulmonary volume decreases.

Fibrosis
Streaky white reticular shadows occur with local fibrosis. Structures are pulled towards the fibrotic region. Generalized fibrosis causes increased lung markings, with either reticular or nodular pattern. Severe generalized fibrosis may cause a honeycomb pattern.

3.2 Radiology

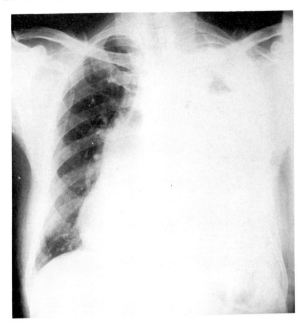

Fig. 29 *Massive left pleural effusion. Note the heart and mediastinum are displaced to the right.*

Widely disseminated shadows (Fig. 30)

Pin point opacities occur in the following conditions:
• fibrosing alveolitis
• haemosiderosis

Opacities 2–4 mm in diameter. These include:
• miliary tuberculosis
• simple coal miners pneumoconiosis
• viral pneumonia
• acute histoplasmosis
• PAN

Opacities 5–8 mm in diameter. These may be caused by:
• sarcoidosis
• multiple metastases (Fig. 31)

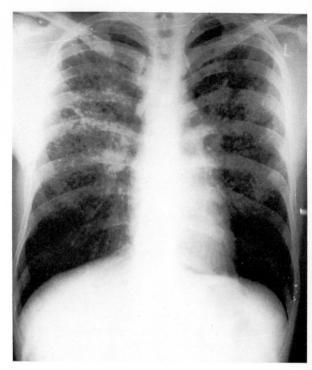

Fig. 30 *Diffuse reticulonodular shadowing in both mid-zones.*

- extrinsic allergic alveolitis
- pulmonary oedema
- tuberculosis

Discrete shadows (Fig. 32)
These shadows within the lungs or mediastinum are usually solitary, but metastases, abscesses and infarcts are often multiple.

The apparently normal X-ray
Even if there are no obvious abnormalities, it is wise to check the X-ray for the following:
- tracheal compression

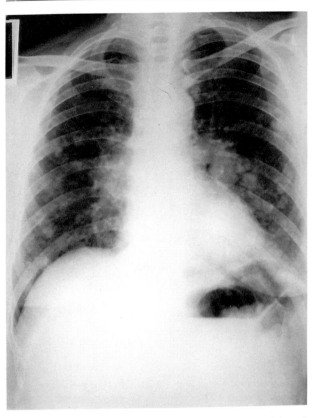

Fig. 31 *Multiple metastases from prostate. Note the nodules of widely differing sizes throughout both lungs.*

- apical pneumothorax
- absent breast shadow (breast cancer)
- secondaries in or fractures of any bones
- rib notching (coarctation of the aorta)
- air under the diaphragm (perforation) (Fig. 33)
- double left heart border (lower lobe collapse)
- fluid level behind heart (achalasia of the cardia)
- paravertebral abscess (TB)

3.0 Investigations

3.2 Radiology

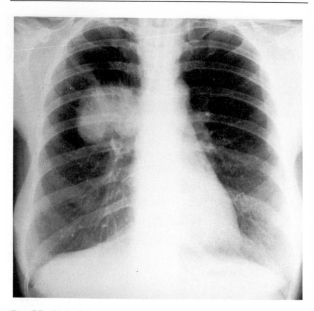

Fig. 32 *Right hilar mass — right upper lobe carcinoma of bronchus.*

Tomography

Tomograms are X-rays 'focused' in one plane of the lung. They may be taken as AP, lateral or oblique views. The focusing is obtained by rotating the film and X-ray source during exposure. AP films are numbered in centimetres from the X-ray plate (the patient's back). The main uses of tomography are as follows:
- for identifying cavitation within lesions (Figs 34 and 35)
- for identifying calcification (suggestive of TB)
- for identifying central tumours: tracheal (Fig. 36), or main bronchial compression
- for clarification of mediastinal and hilar shadows to determine whether they are vascular or glandular
- in seeing whether there are multiple lesions throughout the lungs (i.e. metastases) which are not shown on a plain PA film

3.2 Radiology

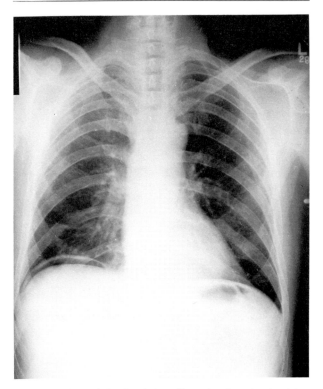

Fig. 33 *Perforated duodenal ulcer. Note the air under the right diaphragm.*

3.2 Radiology

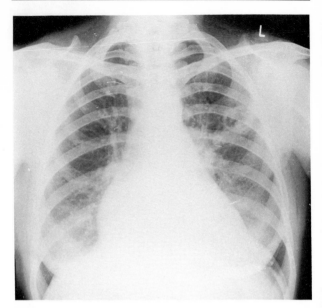

Fig. 34 *Active pulmonary tuberculosis. Note the cavity in the left mid-zone.*

Bronchography (Figs 37 and 38)

The instilling of contrast medium into the bronchial tree is now rare, but is the only definite method of diagnosing bronchiectasis. As it is unpleasant for the patient, the diagnosis is often presumed on other clinical grounds without performing bronchography except if surgery is being considered when one needs to know the extent of the bronchiectasis.

Screening

Fluoroscopic screening is useful for the following:
* checking whether the diaphragm moves (phrenic nerve palsy)
* looking for valvular calcification
* discovering whether a mass is pulsatile, e.g. aortic aneurysm
* use during transbronchial biopsy to try and avoid biopsying

3.2 Radiology

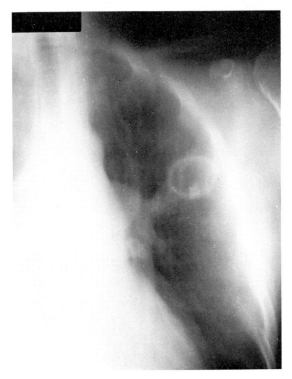

Fig. 35 *Tomogram of Fig. 34 confirming cavitation and showing an area of calcification.*

the pleura, thus avoiding a pneumothorax
- use during percutaneous needle lung biopsies to enable one to biopsy the lesion

Barium studies

Barium swallow is performed to check upon oesophageal indentation or displacement by an enlarged atrium or by mediastinal tumours.

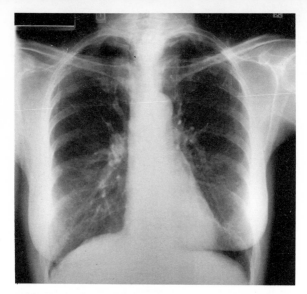

Fig. 36 *Tracheal compression and displacement from a goitre.*

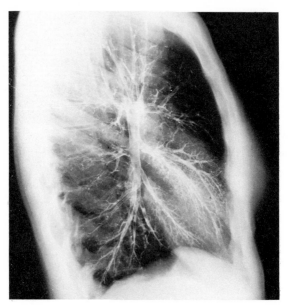

Fig. 37 *Normal bronchogram — lateral view.*

3.2 Radiology

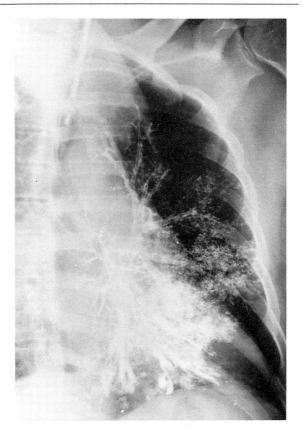

Fig. 38 *Bronchogram showing lingula and left lower lobe bronchiectasis. Note the cylindrical dilatation and pooling of contrast in these regions as opposed to the normal upper lobe.*

Pulmonary angiography (Figs 39 and 40)

This is the definitive procedure in the diagnosis of pulmonary embolism or pulmonary hypertension. However, it carries a small but significant mortality and, therefore, should only be carried out either if all less invasive techniques have been non-diagnostic or in an emergency if surgery is being considered.

77

3.2 Radiology

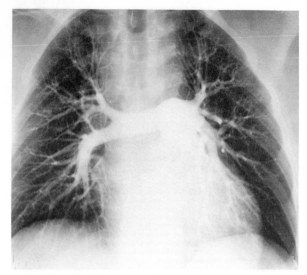

Fig. 39 *Normal pulmonary angiogram.*

Computerized axial tomography (CAT scanning; Fig. 41)

Axial tomograms produce pictures which look like transverse slices through the body viewed from the patient's feet looking towards his head. The two main limitations of this technique in respiratory investigation are its expense (both capital investment and running costs are high), and its unsuitability for very breathless patients because:
• they must be flat
• they have to be able to hold their breath for between 3–20 s (depending on the machine) for each section to be taken.

In respiratory medicine CAT scanning is clinically useful for the following:
• evaluating the mediastinum in patients with lung cancer or lymphoma
• evaluating contralateral lungs in lung cancer
• showing multiple metastases
• finding small primary tumours

3.0 Investigations

3.2 Radiology

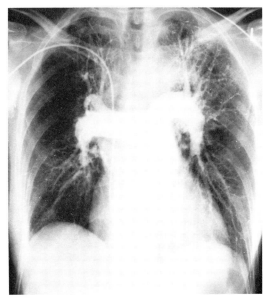

Fig. 40 *Pulmonary angiogram showing occlusion of many major vessels due to pulmonary embolism.*

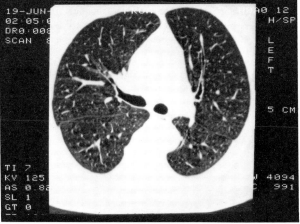

Fig. 41 *Normal CT scan of thorax.*

- showing the extent of interstitial lung diseases and also bullous disease in emphysema
- demonstrating pleural disease
- finding cerebral secondaries
- finding liver secondaries

There is no doubt that a lot of information is obtained by these scans. However, this extra information does not always alter the management of the patient.

3.3 Radioisotope scanning

Lung scans

Radioisotope lung scans are used to diagnose pulmonary emboli. Both ventilation and perfusion scans should be performed because filling defects on perfusion scans are not specific to pulmonary embolism; they are also present in other lung diseases such as emphysema, chronic bronchitis, asthma, fibrosis and pneumonia. In these diseases the ventilation and perfusion scans show congruous defects, whereas in pulmonary embolism they do not. Nevertheless, the interpretation of these scans is often the subject of clinical debate. All that can be said is that a normal perfusion scan virtually excludes a significant pulmonary embolus. In other cases, it may be necessary to revert to pulmonary angiography to prove whether or not the patient has pulmonary vascular disease.

Perfusion lung scans
Microspheres of human serum albumin tagged with ^{131}I (or $^{99}Tc^m$ are injected intravenously). The microspheres are larger (10–50 μm) than the pulmonary capillaries (8 μm) and lodge before breaking up, so that the gamma emission can be counted using a rectilinear scanner. Only 150 000 particles are injected, thus only occluding a representative selection of the 300 million capillaries.

Ventilation lung scans
Either of the gamma-emitting radioactive gases krypton-81^m (if available from a cyclotron) or xenon-133 are inhaled. Krypton-81^m has a much shorter half-life (12.5 s) giving a

3.0 Investigations

3.3 Radioisotope scanning

dynamic scan rather than a volume scan such as those obtained with xenon-133 (half-life 5.3 days). The resolution of the scan is also better with krypton due to the differing energy emission bands of the 2 gases.

Scanning for metastases

Radioisotope (technesium) scans are extensively used in the diagnosis of brain, liver and bone secondaries in patients with bronchial carcinoma. Metastases are relatively more vascular than the surrounding structures, thus they appear as 'hot spots'.

Gallium scans

Gallium-67 citrate (obtained from a cyclotron) is localized in areas of inflammation and in the Kuppfer cells of normal liver. An injection is given followed by a body scan 2–3 days later. The radiation dose is equivalent to a barium enema. The scan is increasingly used for the assessment of the activity of alveolitis in interstitial lung diseases or to find the extent of the granuloma in sarcoidosis. Inflammation of the airways in chronic bronchitis does not give a positive scan.

3.4 Ultrasound

At present, the only established role of ultrasound in chest disease is in the diagnosis and drainage of pleural effusions. Ultrasound is good at localizing and identifying whether a pleural lesion is solid or fluid. This is particularly useful in the aspiration of a loculated pleural effusion. Mediastinal ultrasound via an oesophageal probe is currently being evaluated. Ultrasound is of no value in the diagnosis of other lung lesions because it is dispersed too widely by the air in the lungs, leading to poor echogenicity. Ultrasound is the investigation of choice in excluding liver or adrenal metastases.

3.5   Electrocardiographs (ECGs)

Uses of standard ECG

The main uses of an ECG in respiratory medicine are in the diagnosis of the following complaints.

Myocardial ischaemia or infarction
Presenting as chest pain or shortness of breath (left ventricular failure).

Pulmonary embolism (Fig. 42)
The characteristic SI, QIII, TIII pattern of a pulmonary embolism is rarely seen.

Cor pulmonale
With pulmonary hypertension typically due to chronic obstructive airways disease, the ECG shows a right ventricular hypertrophy and strain pattern (Fig. 43) — P wave is greater than 3 mm (P pulmonale) with right axis deviation. There are tall R waves over the right chest leads and sometimes T wave inversion in these leads.

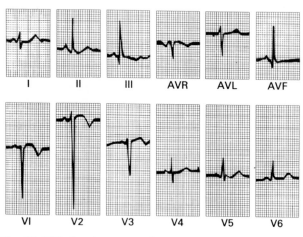

Fig. 42 *ECG showing acute pulmonary embolism. Note the SI QIII TIII pattern together with the inverted T waves in the right chest leads V1 V2.*

3.0 Investigations

3.5 Electrocardiographs (ECGs)

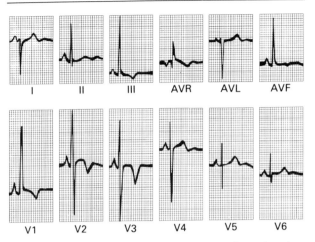

Fig. 43 *ECG showing right ventricular hypertrophy and strain. Note the peaked pulmonale, and the tall R waves with inverted T waves in the right chest leads V1-V3, together with the right axis deviation.*

Pericarditis
This may complicate pneumonia or occur with malignant invasion of the pericardium.

Myocarditis or myocardial infiltration
Myocarditis may occur with viral or atypical pneumonias and infiltration with sarcoidosis.

Rhythm disturbances
Atrial fibrillation is commonly found in patients with ischaemic heart disease, coexisting with chronic lung disease. It may also occur with pericardial infiltration, invasion or inflammation.

24-Hour ECG monitoring

24-hour Holter tape monitoring of the ECG is very useful in the detection of intermittent cardiac dysrhythmias. Although this is often due to myocardial ischaemia, myocardial sarcoidosis may also present with intermittent cardiac arrhythmias.

3.5 Electrocardiographs (ECGs)

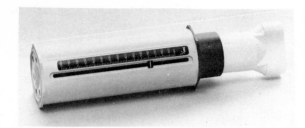

Fig. 44 *Wright peak flow gauge, suitable for use at home.*

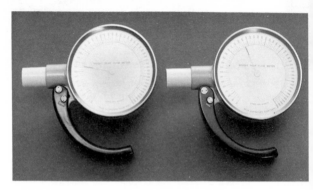

Fig. 45 *Wright peak flow meter before and after bronchodilator, confirming a diagnosis of asthma.*

3.6 Lung function tests

Routine tests

Peak flow and spirometry
Peak expiratory flow rate (PEFR) is measured by a maximal forced expiration through either a Wright's peak flow meter or the cheaper plastic peak flow gauge (Figs 44 and 45). The peak flow correlates well with the forced expiratory volume in one second (FEV_1). Both are used as an estimate of airways calibre. The FEV_1 and forced vital capacity (FVC) are measured from a full forced expiration into a bellows or dry wedge spirometer (Vitalograph, Fig. 46). The FEV_1/FVC ratio gives a good estimate of the severity of airflow obstruction (Fig. 47). Peak

3.6 Lung function tests

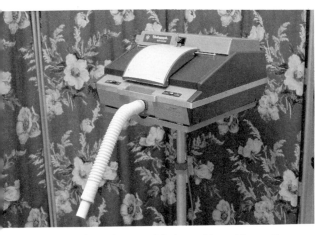

Fig. 46 *Dry wedge spirometer (vitalograph) used for routine spirometry.*

flow rate and spirometry should be repeated 10 minutes after inhaling a β agonist such as salbutamol to assess reversibility. Typical spirograms are shown in Fig. 48.

Lung volumes
Lung volumes, total lung capacity (TLC) and residual volume (RV) may be measured by inspiring a known amount of an inert non-absorbed gas such as helium, the lung volumes can then be calculated from the dilution. A whole-body plethysmograph ('body box') is an alternative way of measuring these volumes (Fig. 49).

Gas transfer
The gas transfer (KCO) across the alveoli is calculated using a respirameter to measure how much of a known amount of carbon monoxide is absorbed from a single inspiration in a standard time — usually a 10 second breath-hold (Fig. 50). The DLCO (transfer factor) is the KCO multiplied by the alveolar volume (VA) simultaneously measured by helium dilution. The KCO and hence DLCO are both affected by the haemoglobin concentration and disturbances of V/Q mismatch.

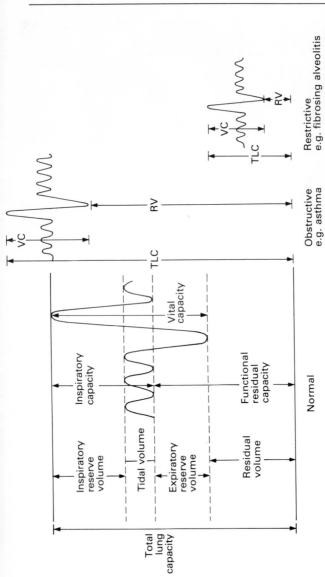

Fig. 17. 8.4 divisions of the total lung capacity, showing changes occurring in obstructive and restrictive ventilatory

3.0 Investigations

3.6 Lung function tests

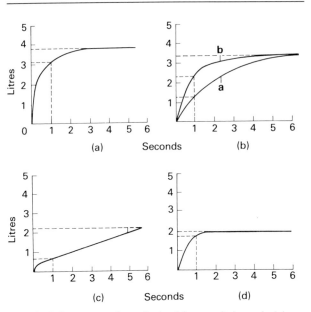

Fig. 48 *Spirogram tracings obtained from a vitalograph. (a) Normal FEV_1 3. 1 l, FVC 3. 8 l, FEV_1/FVC 82%. (b) Obstructive defect (reversible) asthma, **a** before a bronchodilator FEV_1 1. 4 l, FVC 3. 5 l, FEV_1/FVC 40%; **b** after a bronchodilator FEV_1 2.5 l, FVC 3.5 l, FEV_1/FVC 71%. (c) Severe irreversible airways obstruction , chronic bronchitis and emphysema FEV_1 0.5 l, FVC 2.2 l, FEV_1/FVC 23% before and after a bronchodilator. (d) Restrictive defect, fibrosing alveolitis FEV_1 1.8 l, FVC 2.0 l, FEV_1/FVC 90%. No change with bronchodilators.*

Applications of routine lung function tests (Figs 51–53)

Diagnosis
Asthma is diagnosed upon the basis of reversible airways obstruction — an improvement in the PEFR and FEV_1 of 20% after a bronchodilator is diagnostic. The airflow obstruction in chronic bronchitis and emphysema is much less reversible 10–15% maximum increase in FEV_1 after a bronchodilator. The gas transfer is often very low in emphysema due to alveolar destruction.

3.6 Lung function tests

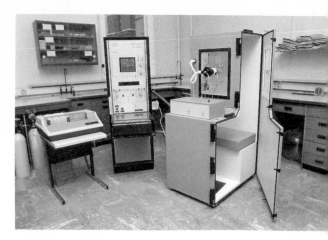

Fig. 49 *Body plethysmograph used for measuring lung volumes and airways resistance and conductance.*

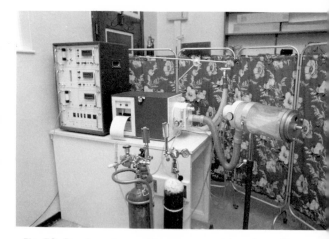

Fig. 50 *Respirameter used to measure gas transfer and lung volumes (helium dilution method).*

3.0 Investigations

3.6 Lung function tests

Table 5 Typical patterns of abnormal lung function tests.

	'Obstructive pattern' (e.g. asthma, chronic bronchitis and emphysema)	'Restrictive pattern' (e.g. acinar lung disease such as fibrosing alveolitis or sarcoidosis)
PEFR	$\downarrow\downarrow$	Normal or $\downarrow$
FEV_1	$\downarrow\downarrow$	$\downarrow\downarrow$
FVC	Normal or $\downarrow$	$\downarrow$
$FEV_1/FVC\%$	$<70\%$	$>80\%$
Gas transfer [KCO and DLCO]	Normal or $\uparrow$ — asthma, $\downarrow$ chronic bronchitis, $\downarrow\downarrow$ emphysema	$\downarrow\downarrow$
TLC	$\uparrow$ Asthma $\uparrow\uparrow$ Emphysema Normal–chronic bronchitis	$\downarrow\downarrow$
RV	$\uparrow\uparrow$	$\downarrow$
Airways resistance	$\uparrow\uparrow$	Normal or $\downarrow$
Conductance	$\downarrow\downarrow$	Normal or $\uparrow$
Response of FEV_1 to β agonists	$>20\%$ = asthma $<20\%$ = chronic bronchitis or emphysema	None

Interstitial disease causes small stiff lungs with impaired gas transfer.

Monitoring therapy
The response to bronchodilators (including steroids) and the control of asthma is best monitored by regular peak flow rates or FEV_1. The effects of therapy upon interstitial lung disease are judged by changes in gas transfer and lung volumes.

Preoperative assessment
Two questions should be asked.
1. Is there any possibility of improving the lung function prior

3.0 Investigations

3.6 Lung function tests

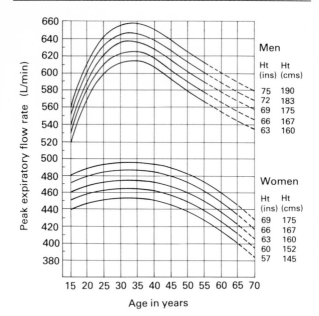

Fig. 51 *Normal values for peak expiratory flow rates according to sex, age and height.*

to anaesthetic? This is often possible in patients with unsuspected asthma or other chronic airflow obstruction. If possible, operation should be delayed until maximal improvement has been obtained.

2. Is the absolute lung function too poor for a general anaesthetic? The problem is not in giving an anaesthetic but in the recovery period, particularly if painful upper abdominal surgery has been performed which is likely to splint the diaphragm leading to hypoventilation and respiratory failure — perhaps necessitating artificial ventilation for a while. Patients with PEFR < 100 l/min or FEV_1 < 1.0 l should be assessed very carefully before a general anaesthetic is given — local anaesthetics should be considered where possible.

3.0 Investigations

3.6 Lung function tests

Thoracic surgery
Lung function tests are essential prior to cardiothoracic surgery, particularly if resection of a lobe or lung is intended (see page 233).

More specialized tests

Resistance and conductance
Airways resistance is measured in a body plethysmograph as is the conductance (GAW) which is the reciprocal of resistance. The slope of conductance plotted against lung volume is specific airways conductance (SGAW). In diseases such as asthma or chronic bronchitis characterized by airways obstruction the resistance is increased and conductance reduced.

Flow volume loops (Figs 54 and 55)
A complete forced respiratory manoeuvre (full expiration followed by a full inspiration, starting at TLC) is performed. Flow rate is plotted against volume (the spirogram is time-plotted against volume). The four main abnormalities of these loops are:
1. a characteristic scalloping of the expiratory portion of the curve in asthma and chronic bronchitis;
2. in emphysema there is relatively well-preserved peak flow with 'early airways collapse' in the expiratory phase;
3. upper airways obstruction is shown by 'cut off' of the inspiratory loop;
4. the last part of the expiratory phase of the flow volume loop (the flow rates at low lung volumes) may be the earliest detectable abnormalities with small airways disease — such as in smokers.

Exercise tests

Several types are available: each is performed with a different purpose in mind. Exercise tests should always be performed with a doctor present and full resuscitation equipment should be immediately available.

Tests to assess limitation and improvement after therapy
The distance the patient walks on the flat in 12 minutes is measured. This gives a measure of exercise tolerance.

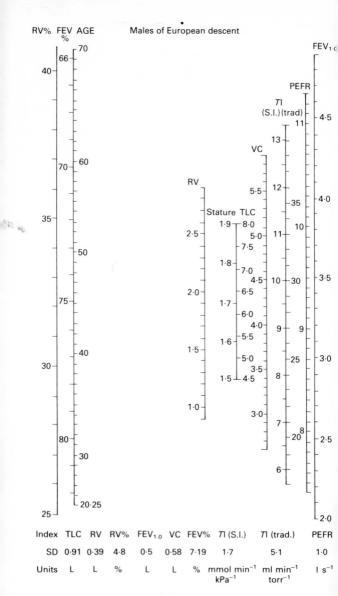

Males of European descent

Index	TLC	RV	RV%	FEV$_{1.0}$	VC	FEV%	TI (S.I.)	TI (trad.)	PEFR
SD	0.91	0.39	4.8	0.5	0.58	7.19	1.7	5.1	1.0
Units	L	L	%	L	L	%	mmol min^{-1} kPa^{-1}	ml min^{-1} torr^{-1}	l s^{-1}

(a)

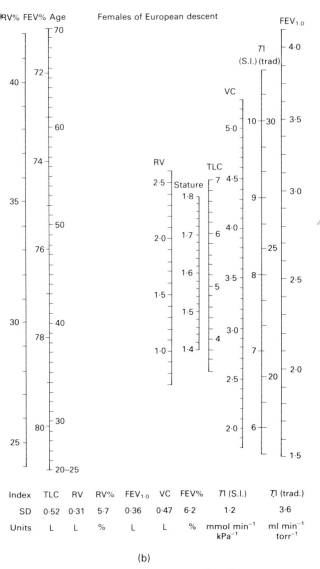

Fig. 52 (a) and (b) Normal values for lung function tests according to age, sex and height in patients of European descent.

93

3.0 Investigations

3.6 Lung function tests

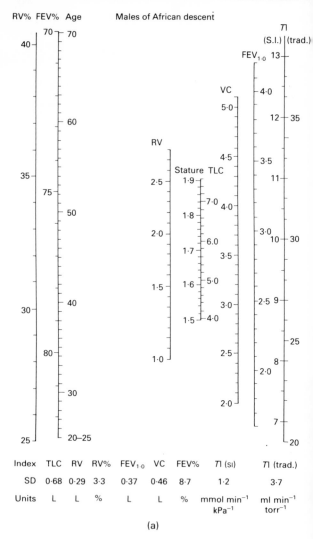

Index	TLC	RV	RV%	FEV$_{1.0}$	VC	FEV%	Tl (SI)	Tl (trad.)
SD	0.68	0.29	3.3	0.37	0.46	8.7	1.2	3.7
Units	L	L	%	L	L	%	mmol min^{-1} kPa^{-1}	ml min^{-1} torr^{-1}

(a)

Fig. 53 *(a) and (b) Normal values for lung function tests according to age, sex and height in patients of African descent.*

3.6 Lung function tests

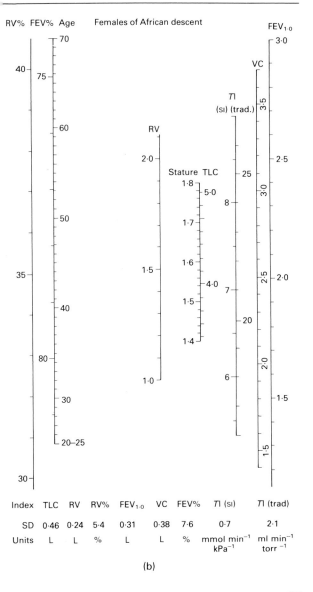

Index	TLC	RV	RV%	FEV$_{1.0}$	VC	FEV%	Tl (SI)	Tl (trad)
SD	0·46	0·24	5·4	0·31	0·38	7·6	0·7	2·1
Units	L	L	%	L	L	%	mmol min^{-1} kPa^{-1}	ml min^{-1} torr^{-1}

(b)

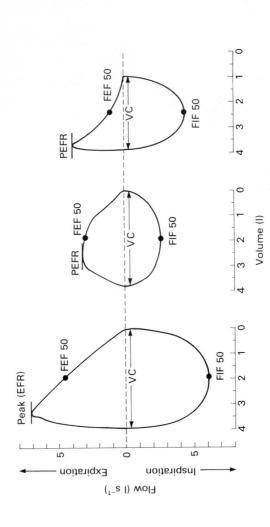

Fig. 54 Flow volume loops. (a) Normal. (b) Extrathoracic upper airways obstruction — tracheal stenosis. (c) Intrathoracic airways obstruction — asthma.

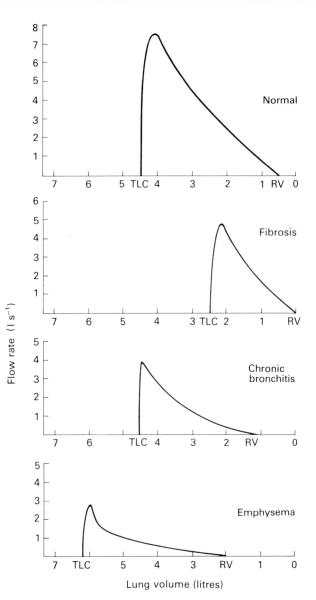

Fig. 55 *Flow volume loops to show changes in common diseases and accompanying changes in lung volumes at which they occur.*

3.6 Lung function tests

It may be repeated after therapy to give objective evidence of improvement. It is important to realize that there is a 'learning curve' in that the patient's performance improves with the first three or four walks without any therapy.

Tests to induce bronchospasm

The peak flow rate (or FEV_1) is recorded before running up and down the stairs for 5 minutes, then immediately on completion of exercise and at 5-minute intervals up to ½ hour. A fall of greater than 20% from baseline indicates exercise-induced asthma (Fig. 56). The test can be repeated after sodium cromoglycate, salbutamol, or ipratropium pre-treatment to assess response to therapy. The same information can often be obtained by hyperventilation or challenge with histamine or cold air rather than exercise.

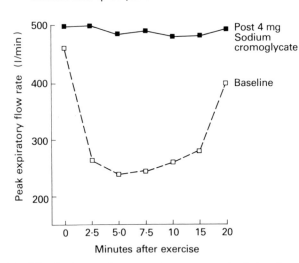

Exercise test: ♀ 21 years

Fig. 56 *Simple exercise test to diagnose exercise-induced asthma. Baseline the patient runs, following which her peak flow is measured, this has dropped from 460 l/min to 240 l/m at 5 min, thus confirming the diagnosis. The following day the patient underwent the same test having been treated with sodium cromoglycate 20 min before the test. The bronchoconstriction was completely prevented.*

3.0 Investigations

3.6 Lung function tests

Formal exercise testing
Ventilation, heart rate, oxygen uptake and saturation are measured at various work rates, either on a bicycle ergometer or treadmill. This is particularly useful in evaluating the symptom of breathlessness on exertion if routine clinical examination and other tests have failed to yield a diagnosis. Recurrent thrombo-embolism is often an example of such a problem.

3.7 Blood gases (Figs 57–59)

Measurement

Heparinized blood samples are taken from the radial, brachial or

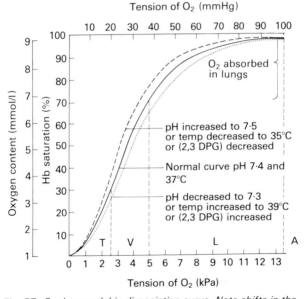

Fig. 57 *Oxyhaemoglobin dissociation curve. Note shifts in the curve due to changes in pH, temperature and 2, 3 DPG. Note that the oxygen-carrying capacity of blood does not fall much until there has been a considerable reduction in the* Pao_2*. T = tissues; L = lungs; V = venous; A = arterial.*

3.0 Investigations

3.7 Blood gases

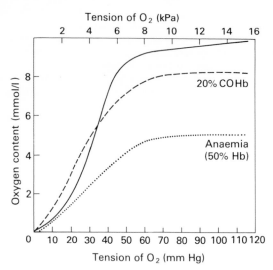

Fig. 58 *Oxyhaemoglobin dissociation curve showing the effects of anaemia and heavy smoking upon oxygen carriage.*

femoral arteries taking care to avoid introducing air bubbles into the syringe. The Pao_2, $Paco_2$ and pH are measured rapidly by an automated analyser.

At the bedside, $Paco_2$ can also be measured by the rebreathing method.
1. The patient breaths for 1½ minutes into a 1.5 litre bag.
2. He rests for 2 minutes.
3. He then rebreathes for 5 breaths or 20 seconds, whichever is longer.
4. The CO_2 content can now be measured by Haldane or other analyser
   - % CO_2 × barometric pressure = Pco_2 (venous)
   - venous Pco_2 − 6 = arterial Pco_2 (mmHg)

Oxygen content and hence saturation may be measured directly by the Van Slyke manometric method or by spectrophotometry. Ear oximetry is a useful method for measuring changes in the oxygen saturation by non-invasive means.

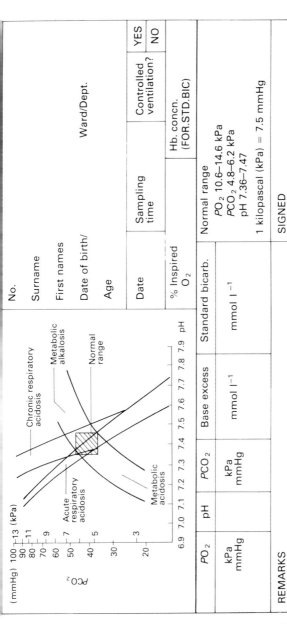

Fig. 59 Report form for blood gas analysis showing normal ranges and shifts with acid base disturbances.

101

3.0 Investigations

3.7 Blood gases

Transcutaneous electrodes are also available for measuring $T_cP_{O_2}$, $T_cP_{CO_2}$ and pH. However, transcutaneous values are very dependent upon blood pressure and tissue perfusion.

Interpretation

Low Pa_{O_2}
Hypoxia occurs for one or more of the following reasons:
- ventilation/perfusion (V/Q) mismatch
- hypoventilation
- abnormal diffusion

Table 6 Typical patterns of blood gas abnormalities.

	Pa_{O_2}	Pa_{CO_2}	Reason
Asthma — Mild	↓	↓	V/Q mismatch with hyperventilation
— Moderate	↓↓	Normal	worsening airways obstruction
— Severe	↓↓↓	↑	leading to hypoventilation
Chronic bronchitis	↓↓	↑	V/Q mismatch and hypoventilation
Emphysema	Normal or ↓	↓	V/Q mismatch and hyperventilation
Fibrosing alveolitis Left ventricular failure or pulmonary embolus	↓↓	↓ or Normal	V/Q mismatch and hyperventilation Abnormal diffusion
Hysterical hyperventilation	Normal	↓	Hyperventilation — normal lungs
Type I Respiratory failure	↓↓↓	Normal	V/Q mismatch
Type II Respiratory failure	↓↓↓	↑↑	Hypoventilation and V/Q mismatch

---

• right to left cardiac shunts

V/Q mismatch is by far the most common cause.

Abnormal $Paco_2$
The $Paco_2$ is directly related to alveolar ventilation. V/Q mismatch has much less effect. In most clinical situations:
• low $Paco_2$ = hyperventilation
• high $Paco_2$ = hypoventilation

Acid base balance

• $CO_2 + H_2O \rightleftharpoons H_2CO_3 \rightleftharpoons H^+ + HCO_3^-$
• $pH = pK_1 + \log \dfrac{(HCO_3^-)}{(H_2CO_3)}$ (Henderson-Hasselbalch)

CO_2 excretion is rapidly regulated by the *lungs* whereas H^+ and HCO_3^- are slowly controlled by the kidney.

Respiratory acidosis
Hypoventilation causes carbon dioxide retention and hence a sharp increase in H_2CO_3 and H^+, and thus a decrease in pH. A respiratory acidosis ensues. The bicarbonate is normal in an acute respiratory acidosis, but has time to rise in a chronic respiratory acidosis.

Metabolic acidosis
With increased tissue H^+ production, this is buffered by HCO_3^- which is 'mopped up' by increasing H_2CO_3 production. More carbon dioxide is produced and rapidly 'blown off' via the lungs. Metabolic acidosis is, therefore, recognized primarily by a fall in HCO_3^-. The patient hyperventilates to eliminate the extra CO_2 produced.

Respiratory alkalosis
Hyperventilation causes carbon dioxide excretion to be increased, hence a fall in H_2CO_3 and H^+ occurs, with consequent rise in the pH. In an acute respiratory alkalosis the HCO_3^- remains relatively constant, only in a chronic situation will it tend to fall when the kidney has had time to compensate.

Metabolic alkalosis
Either excessive loss of H^+ as in persistent vomiting or excess

ingestion of alkalis lead to this rare situation. It is often associated with hypokalaemia.

3.8 Skin tests

Allergy testing (Figs 60 and 61)

Skin prick tests bear a good correlation with specific IgE antibody. Antigen reacts with specific IgE reaginic antibody in a local type 1 hypersensitivity reaction. The tests are performed on the volar aspect of the forearm with some of the numerous commercially available antigen solutions. If positive, a weal and flare reaction is seen within 10–20 minutes (due to histamine release from the sensitized mast cells). The reaction fades in

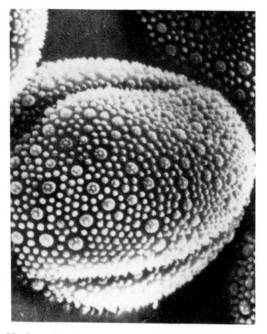

Fig. 60 *Scanning electron micrograph (SEM) of silver birch pollen.*

3.8 Skin tests

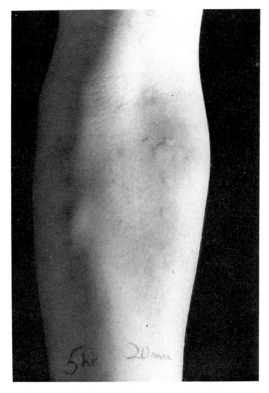

Fig. 61 *Forearm showing positive allergy skin prick tests.*

1–1½ hours. Common antigens which are used are as follows:

- house dust
- house dust mite
- grass pollens
- tree pollens
- cat fur
- dog fur
- feathers
- aspergillus

Skin prick tests are very safe and easy to perform, but
extremely rarely bronchospasm may be induced and hence a

3.8   Skin tests

bronchodilator should always be available. Intradermal tests add little information and are more hazardous. Bronchial provocation tests are potentially even more hazardous and should only be performed as an in-patient procedure with full resuscitation equipment nearby. They should be done using one antigen at a time. The rationale for bronchial provocation testing is that not all the antigens which give positive skin tests are necessarily responsible for inducing asthma attacks.

The 2 main uses of skin tests are in identifying avoidable allergens and identifying those asthmatics of all ages who are likely to respond to disodium cromoglycate, a drug which is less likely to aid skin-test-negative patients. However, as the range of antigens is infinite, a negative reaction to a few selected allergens does not necessarily mean that there is not an allergic cause for the patient's asthma. The patient's history is most important in identifying possible allergic causes.

Drugs and allergy skin tests
- antihistamines ⎫
- β-agonist therapy ⎭ reduce immediate skin test reaction
- steroids — no effect on the immediate responses

Tuberculin testing

Types
There are three commonly used tuberculin tests.

Mantoux test.   0.1 ml old tuberculin 1:10 000 (1 TU) or 1:1000 (10 TU) is injected intradermally into the volar surface of the forearm (Fig. 62). The diameter of induration is measured at 48–72 hours. The erythema is ignored. 10 mm of induration is a positive test (Fig. 63). Testing starts with the most dilute solution.

Heaf test.   Using a special injection gun (Figs 64 and 65) 6 needles puncture the skin to 2 mm depth, through a drop of purified protein derivative (PPD) 2 mg/ml. The test is read after 3–7 days.
Grade I   — 4 separate papules
Grade II   — confluent ring of induration
Grade III   — indurated disc spreading outwards
Grade IV   — plateau of induration of over 10 mm in diameter

3.0 Investigations

3.8 Skin tests

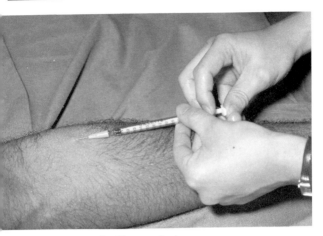

Fig. 62 *Insertion of a Mantoux test.*

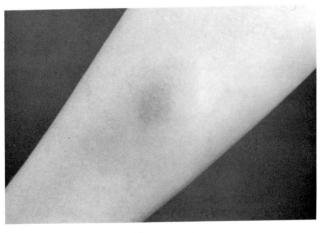

Fig. 63 *Strongly positive Mantoux test.*

Tine test. Each tine unit consists of a stainless steel disc with 4 prongs (tines) attached to a plastic handle (Fig. 66). The tines are covered with dried old tuberculin. The reactivity is equivalent to a Mantoux test of 5 TU.

3.8 Skin tests

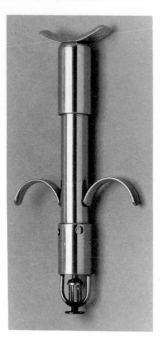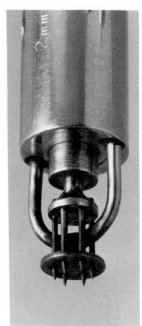

Fig. 64 *(Left) Heaf test gun showing prongs withdrawn.*

Fig. 65 *(Right) Heaf test gun showing prongs extended.*

The disc is pressed firmly onto the patient's forearm for 1 second so that 4 visible puncture marks can be seen.

The test is read after 48–72 hours. A reaction of 5 mm or more around one or more puncture sites is taken as positive. 2–4 mm is taken as doubtful. Less than 2 mm is negative.

Interpretation

Most patients with active TB respond to 10 TU in the Mantoux or have a Heaf grade III or IV response. Some very ill patients with TB including the old or immunosuppressed only respond to 100 TU. A negative Mantoux test 1:100 (100 TU) makes TB very unlikely, but not impossible as negative tests have been recorded in some very ill patients with active disease. A

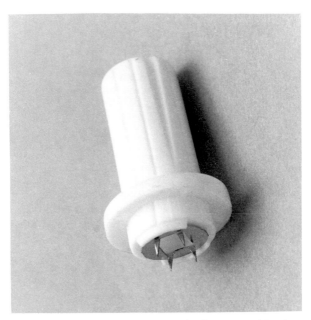

Fig. 66 *Tine test applicator showing the four prongs (tines).*

positive test is never diagnostic of active disease in the UK
because the patient may also either have had the disease
previously and developed immunity or have been immunized
with the Bacille Calmette-Guérin (BCG) vaccination.

Kveim testing

Kveim saline suspension is made from a homogenate of human
sarcoid spleen or lymph nodes. The test is performed by
injecting 0.1–0.2 ml into the skin of the forearm. The site is
marked with an adjacent dot of pelican ink. Within a month a
purplish red nodule may appear in a positive test. Whether or
not this appears, a core biopsy of skin is taken after 4–6 weeks
using a Hayes-Martin drill. A positive test is one with epithelioid
granuloma formation, care should be taken to exclude the
possibility of confusing this with a foreign body granuloma
reaction.

3.0 Investigations

3.8 Skin tests

Interpretation
Careful validation of Kveim suspension is very important.
- A positive test is virtually diagnostic of sarcoidosis
- Overall in sarcoidosis the Kveim test is positive in 75% of patients
- There is a higher positive yield (up to 90%) in patients with early active sarcoidosis, hilar adenopathy and erythema nodosum

3.9 Bronchoscopy

Fibreoptic bronchoscopy is well tolerated under a premedication and local anaesthesia. Despite this and despite the wider range of view and biopsy afforded by the fibreoptic instrument compared with the rigid scope there is little, if any, evidence to suggest that lung cancer is being diagnosed any earlier.

Indications

The main indications are to investigate:
- hilar or perihilar masses seen on chest X-ray
- slowly resolving pneumonia — (1) to exclude a neoplasm, (2) to obtain bacteriological samples, and (3) to exclude the inhalation of a foreign body
- unexplained haemoptysis — to localize the site of bleeding and find the cause
- interstitial lung disease — transbronchial biopsy and bronchoalveolar lavage

or to treat:
- by aspiration of mucus plugs which are causing lobar collapse (i.e. post-operative or on intensive care units; Figs 68 and 69)

Rigid bronchoscopy is preferable in the following circumstances:
- investigation and treatment of *profuse* haemoptysis
- extraction of foreign bodies and mucus plugs (Fig. 70)
- assessment of bronchial mobility for immediate pre-operative appraisal in lung cancer

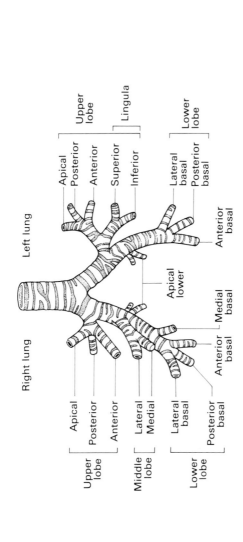

Fig. 67 The anatomy of the tracheobronchial tree. Two lobes on the left (approximately 45% of total lung volume) and three lobes on the right (approximately 55% of total lung volume).

3.9 Bronchoscopy

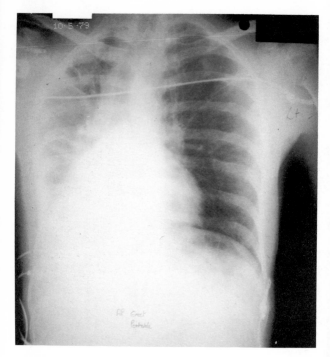

Fig. 68 *Patient with a collapsed right lower lobe due to a mucus plug following an anaesthetic.*

Preparation (Figs 71–4)

- Check that the patient has adequate lung function (peak flow rate > 100 l/min) to receive a premedication; otherwise use local anaesthetic alone
- Check the patient is not allergic to drugs, in particular opiates and local anaesthetics
- Check Hepatitis B antigen status of patient
- Check HTLV III antibody status
- Check blood clotting is normal
- Give the patient oxygen 2 l/min via the other nostril

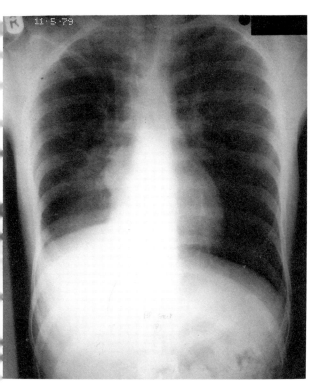

Fig. 69 *The same patient as shown in Fig. 68 12 hours after the extraction of the mucus plug using a fibreoptic bronchoscope.*

Premedication and local anaesthesia

The two commonly used premedications are mixtures of either:

Atropine 0.6 mg
+
Diazepam 5–10 mg   } i.v. at the time of bronchoscopy
+
Fentanyl 50–100 μg

3.9   Bronchoscopy

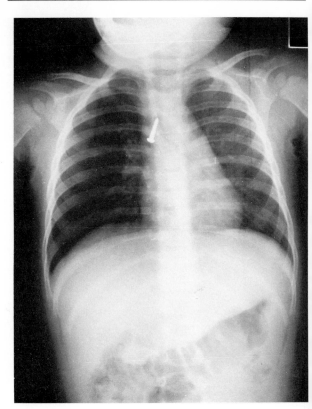

Fig. 70 *Foreign body (screw) in the right main bronchus of a child.*

or

Omnopon 20 mg
+
Scopolamine 0.4 mg } i.m. 30 minutes prior to the bronchoscopy

Lignocaine is used as local anaesthetic-10% spray for the nose and the oropharynx, 2 ml 4% for the larynx and 2 ml 2% for each side of the bronchial tree.

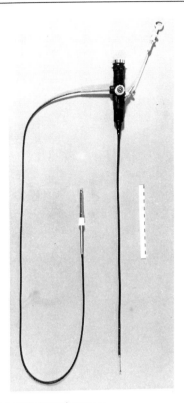

Fig. 71 *Fibreoptic bronchoscope.*

Procedure (Figs 75–8)

The bronchoscope is passed nasally. The larynx is inspected, in particular to assess the mobility of the vocal cords. The position, size and extent of spread of any lesions within the tracheobronchial tree are noted. Mucus is extracted and sent for culture (including mycobacteria) and cytology in all cases. Any mucosal abnormalities should be brushed for cytology and then biopsied.

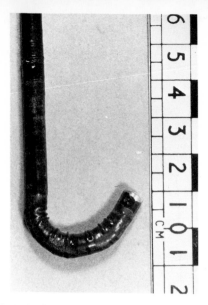

Fig. 72 *End of a fibreoptic bronchoscope showing the size and flexibility.*

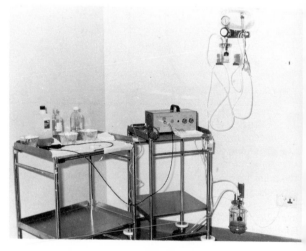

Fig. 73 *General preparation and requirements for fibreoptic bronchoscopy. Note light source, oxygen, suction, antiseptics and local anaesthetics.*

3.9 Bronchoscopy

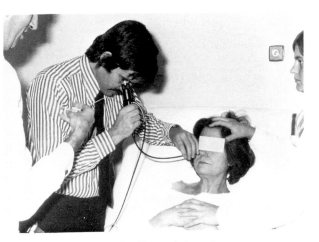

Fig. 74 *Patient undergoing fibreoptic bronchoscopy.*

Results

Typical overall success rates in the diagnosis of malignant
lesions are: biopsy, 70%; brushings, 80%. By comparison,
rigid bronchoscopy has a 50% yield.

Complications

Respiratory depression (hypoxaemia)
This is caused by the premedication rather than the
bronchoscopy itself. Oxygen should be given during the
bronchoscopy. Naloxone should be readily available to reverse
the effects of the opiates given as premedication.

Bleeding
Bleeding is rarely troublesome, but always warn the patient to
expect a little haemoptysis for the day following the procedure
if a biopsy has been taken.

3.9   Bronchoscopy

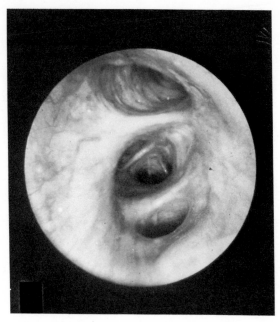

Fig. 75 *View of normal bronchi through a bronchoscope.*

Pneumothorax
This follows a transbronchial biopsy if the pleural surface of the lung has been punctured. It is for this reason that X-ray screening of the procedure is desirable. Pneumothoraces are small and exceedingly rarely require active intervention.

3.10   Bronchoalveolar lavage

This technique is increasingly being used for research and for monitoring the activity of the alveolitis in sarcoidosis and cryptogenic fibrosing alveolitis.

3.10   Bronchoalveolar lavage

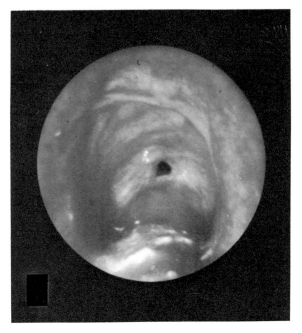

Fig. 76 *Tracheal stenosis at the level of a previous tracheostomy.*

Procedure

1. Check pulmonary function is adequate ($FEV_1 > 1.0$, $Pa_{O_2} > 75$ mmHg).
2. Give supplementary oxygen via nasal cannula.
3. Perform fibreoptic bronchoscopy and wedge bronchoscope into the chosen segmental orifice, usually medial segment of lower lobe.
4. Instil 3×60 ml aliquots of warmed (37 °C) buffered 0.9% saline in and recover with gentle suction. Lavage up to 2 different sites.

3.10 Bronchoalveolar lavage

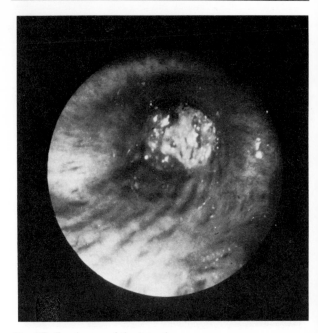

Fig. 77 *Carcinoma of the bronchus.*

Typical results

	Returned volume	Total cell number	Macro-phages (%)	Lympho-cytes (%)	Neutro-phils (%)
Non-smokers	30–60%	$10-22 \times 10^6$	80–90	5–10	2–12
Smokers	30–60%	$20-30 \times 10^6$	70–90	5–15	10–20
Cryptogenic fibrosing alveolitis	30–60%	$25-35 \times 10^6$	40–80	7–10	5–50
Inactive sarcoidosis	30–60%	$20-30 \times 10^6$	70–90	5–25	5–10
Active sarcoidosis	30–60%	$20-30 \times 10^6$	35–50	25–65	5–10

3.10   Bronchoalveolar lavage

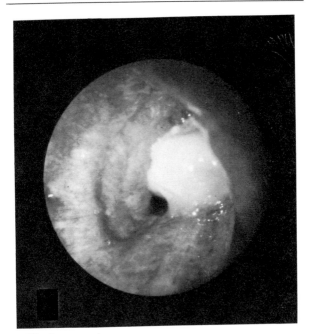

Fig. 78   *A mucus plug.*

There is debate about the correlation between the cell counts obtained by lavage and tissue cell counts from open lung biopsy sections. The alteration of cell numbers due to smoking and chronic bronchitis makes the results difficult to interpret when these conditions co-exist with sarcoidosis, cryptogenic fibrosing alveolitis or other causes of alveolitis.

Complications

- Hypoxia — $Pa{o_2}$ usually falls 5–10 mmHg — if supplementary O_2 is not given greater falls may occur
- Fever — transient slight fever after 12–24 hours is common
- X-ray shadow — a transient shadow is common until the excess lavage fluid is absorbed
- Infection (rare)

3.11 Lung biopsy techniques

Biopsies are required from three kinds of lesion
- central lesions visible through a bronchoscope
- solid peripheral masses beyond bronchoscopic view — percutaneous needle biopsy or transbronchial or open lung biopsy are needed
- interstitial lung disease — transbronchial, drill or open biopsy are indicated

For all lung biopsies check the blood clotting (platelet count and prothrombin time), cross-match 2 units of blood, check hepatitis B and HTLV III antibody status.

Transbronchial lung biopsy (Fig. 79)

If a fibreoptic bronchoscopy is performed under X-ray screening, brushings, aspirates and biopsies can sometimes be obtained from discrete lesions beyond direct vision although a percutaneous needle biopsy is usually needed. With acinar lung disease, multiple biopsies (4 or 5) are taken from *one* lung using X-ray screening so that one avoids the pleura. After the procedure, the patient is X-rayed to exclude a pneumothorax and should rest in bed for 24 hours with regular blood pressure and pulse checks, initially every half an hour.

Complications
- Pneumothorax ⎫ very rarely serious
- Haemorrhage ⎭

Percutaneous needle biopsies

Discrete lesions may be needled directly under X-ray screening through the chest wall using a local anaesthetic. A variety of fine needles are available through which one can aspirate cells.

Precautions
- Pneumothorax ⎫ more frequent than with transbronchial
- Haemorrhage ⎭ biopsies but rarely serious
- Air embolism — exceedingly rare

3.11 Lung biopsy techniques

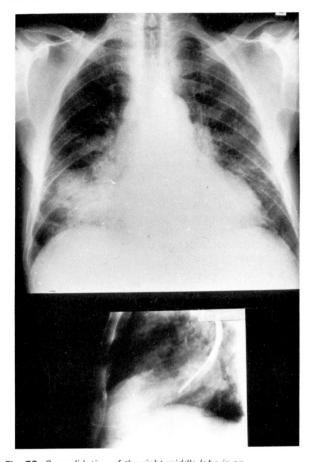

Fig. 79 *Consolidation of the right middle lobe in an immunosuppressed patient. The lateral view shows a transbronchial biopsy being taken through the fibreoptic bronchoscope.*

Compressed air percutaneous drill biopsy

The percutaneous drill biopsy technique obtains larger specimens than the transbronchial biopsy. It is carried out under local anaesthesia exclusively to investigate interstitial lung disease. This technique is not suitable for performing biopsies on discrete masses. The precautions and complications are the same as for other percutaneous needle biopsies. X-ray screening is not used. Because the biopsy is larger the complications are greater — in particular pneumothorax is common.

Open lung biopsy

If other biopsy techniques fail to provide material of diagnostic quality, then thoracotomy and biopsy of the lung are required, if the patient is fit enough.

3.12 Other surgical diagnostic procedures

Surgical diagnostic procedures performed under general anaesthesia include the following.

Mediastinoscopy and mediastinotomy

These are particularly useful to take biopsies of lymph nodes to diagnose tuberculosis, sarcoidosis, lymphoma or cancer, or to explore any other mediastinal tumour.

Lymph node biopsy

Biopsies of the cervical, scalene or other palpable nodes may be performed for the same reasons as mediastinal nodes. Clearly, if these more accessible nodes are pathologically enlarged it is much safer to biopsy them than to explore the mediastinum.

Thoracoscopy

When 'blind' needle biopsies of the pleura have failed to provide a diagnosis, thoracoscopy is useful in obtaining pleural biopsies under direct vision. At the same time pleural fluid can be drained and a pleurodesis performed if required.

3.13   Immunological tests

Immunoglobulins

Normal values
- IgG 5–15 g/l
- IgM 0.5–1.5 g/l
- IgA 1.5–4.5 g/l
- IgE 0.5–5.0 mg/l

Abnormalities

Non-specific rises in serum immunoglobulin levels may be found in the following diseases which affect the lungs:

- sarcoidosis
- cryptogenic fibrosing alveolitis
- systemic lupus erythematosus (SLE)
- silicosis
- extrinsic allergic alveolitis
- bronchiectasis

Low levels of serum immunoglobulins are found in some patients with recurrent chest infections and bronchiectasis. In particular, sputum and serum IgA levels should be measured in these patients.

Raised total IgE levels are also non-specific and may be associated with:

- asthma
- aspergillosis
- helminth infestations
- tropical eosinophilia

Specific IgE antibodies

Numerous methods are available to measure specific IgE antibody. The commonest are:

- radioimmunosorbent test (RIST)
- radioallergosorbent test (RAST)
- enzyme-linked immunosorbent assay (ELISA)

Each of these is used to identify specific IgE antibody to antigens, e.g. pollen, house dust mite, food antigens. There is good correlation between RAST tests and immediate skin tests, but skin tests are quicker and cheaper.

Precipitins

Serum IgG precipitins are looked for in extrinsic allergic alveolitis. The commonest antigens used are micropolyspora faeni (in farmer's lung) and the proteins in avian droppings (in bird fancier's lung). Precipitins to the particular antigen are found in up to 85% of patients affected with the relevant disease, but they can be found in up to 20% of healthy people who have contact with the antigen but no disease. Thus, a negative test is evidence against the diagnosis but a positive test is not diagnostic.

Circulating immune complexes

Several different techniques are used to detect the presence of circulating immune complexes. The two commonest are the Cl_q binding and the polyethyleneglycol (PEG) precipitation methods. Using these methods, circulating complexes have been described in many respiratory diseases, including:
- SLE
- polyarteritis nodosum
- cryptogenic fibrosing alveolitis
- sarcoidosis
- tuberculosis
- cystic fibrosis

The presence of immune complexes is, therefore, not diagnostically useful.

Complement

Complement levels as judged by C_3 levels or total haemolytic complement (CH_{50}) are frequently requested in the investigation of interstitial lung disease. Again, changes are non-specific and non-diagnostic. Elevated complement levels are often found in:
- sarcoidosis
- rheumatoid arthritis

- cryptogenic fibrosing alveolitis
- chronic inflammation

Diminished complement levels are found in:
- SLE
- angio-oedema

Congenital complement deficiency is one of the conditions which leads to recurrent respiratory infections.

C_1 esterase inhibitor deficiency is the specific enzyme deficiency in hereditary angio-oedema, and, therefore, the C_1 esterase inhibitor activity should be checked by functional or immunological assay if the history suggests the possibility of this diagnosis.

Antinuclear antibodies (ANF) and rheumatoid factor

Antinuclear antibody titres of 1:10 or greater, and rheumatoid factor of 1:32 or greater, are found in about 5% of the general population. They are also found in many patients with chest disease other than in SLE and rheumatoid arthritis. They are rarely of diagnostic help.

	ANF(%)	Rheumatoid factor(%)
SLE	100	40
fibrosing alveolitis	40	30
rheumatoid arthritis with fibrosing alveolitis	45	70
systemic sclerosis and fibrosing alveolitis	70	0
sarcoidosis	15	5
silicosis	45	10
asbestosis	25	25
carcinoma bronchus	15	5
chronic bronchitis	20	20
intrinsic asthma	25	5
extrinsic asthma	15	15

Specific reactivity to double-stranded DNA is only usual in SLE. Single-stranded DNA antibodies are common in all the listed conditions except asthma.

3.0 Investigations

3.13 Immunological tests

Cellular immunology

Abnormalities in the routine differential white blood cell count occur in the following situations.

Neutrophils
These are often increased in number during bacterial infection (e.g. pneumonia), during steroid therapy, or if under stress.

Eosinophils
An increased eosinophil count is observed in some cases of:
- asthma — more frequently in extrinsic than intrinsic
- pulmonary eosinophilia
- drug therapy, e.g. PAS, isoniazid, penicillin
- lymphoma

Lymphocytes
These are increased in viral infections; they are reduced in number with steroid therapy and in sarcoidosis or AIDS.

Lymphocyte subpopulations
At present, lymphocyte subpopulations are of research interest only. Using monoclonal antibodies it is possible to identify T cells and divide them into the T_4 (helper) and T_8 (suppressor) cells. B cells may also be counted. In sarcoidosis there is an increase in the B cells and suppressor T cells in peripheral blood. In AIDS there are reduced helper T cells.

Lymphocyte function
In-vivo lymphocyte function is tested by a variety of specific delayed hypersensitivity diagnostic skin tests. The Mantoux test is the classic example, others include Histoplasmin. In-vivo reactivity to ubiquitous antigens such as candida and mumps or the hapten dinitrochlorobenzene (DNCB) are general tests of lymphocyte reactivity because over 90% of the population should respond similarly. In-vitro lymphocyte function can be tested by transformation to antigens such as PPD, or the plant lectins phytohaemagglutinin (PHA) or Conconavalin A (ConA). Lymphocyte function is typically impaired in sarcoidosis and malignant disease. Although widely used in research these in-vitro tests are rarely applied clinically in respiratory disease.

4.0 Common X-ray presentations

4.1 Pleural effusion

Following inflammation, irritation or neoplastic invasion of the pleura, there is exudation of fluid (protein > 30 g/l) which, if it accumulates in the pleural cavity faster than it can be reabsorbed, develops into a pleural effusion. In conditions with impaired drainage of the pleural space due to raised venous pressure, fluid retention or a low serum albumin, there is transudation of fluid (protein content < 30 g/l).

Causes

Common causes of pleural effusions are as follows.

Transudate (protein < 30 g/l)
- Left ventricular failure — by far the commonest cause
- Hypoproteinaemia — hepatic cirrhosis or the nephrotic syndrome
- Constrictive pericarditis
- Meig's syndrome (ovarian fibroma)

Exudate (protein > 30 g/l)
- Malignancy — either direct spread or metastases from a bronchial neoplasm or metastatic spread from other primaries, such as breast, pancreas, kidney, gastrointestinal tract, uterus, ovary, testis and lymphoma, all these effusions often contain blood
- Tuberculosis
- Post-pneumonic — often bacterial in origin; effusion is usually small
- Pulmonary infarction following pulmonary embolism — usually blood-stained and small
- Connective tissue disorders — rheumatoid arthritis, SLE
- Mesothelioma — primary malignancy of the pleura
- Pancreatitis
- Drugs — methysergide, practolol, oxprenolol

Haemothorax
Blood may collect in the pleural cavity secondary to one of three causes:
- trauma — blunt or penetrating injuries
- malignancy ⎫ effusion is usually blood-
- pulmonary infarction ⎭ stained rather than pure blood

131

4.1 Pleural effusion

Empyema
Pus in the pleural space occurs with:
- bacterial pneumonia — most commonly
- TB
- subphrenic abscess
- ruptured oesophagus
- penetrating chest wounds
- post-surgery
- after chest aspiration if strict aseptic technique has not been used

Chylothorax
This is a rare condition, involving leakage of lymph, especially from the thoracic duct, into the pleural cavity. It is usually associated with either neoplastic conditions (e.g. bronchial carcinoma or lymphoma) or trauma.

Clinical features

The commonest symptom due to a pleural effusion is breathlessness, the severity depending upon the volume of fluid and the reserve of the rest of the lungs. Pleuritic pain may also occur, usually in the early stages. Physical signs on the side of a pleural effusion include:
- reduced movement
- stony dull percussion note
- decreased or absent breath sounds
- bronchial breathing at the upper level of the fluid

Investigations

Plain chest X-ray
There must be about 300 ml of fluid in the pleural space for it to be seen on a plain PA chest X-ray and 500 ml or more for it to be detected clinically (Figs 80–2). The upper level of an effusion depends upon gravity. Thus if there is any doubt as to whether a shadow on the PA X-ray is caused by fluid, a film taken with the patient lying on his side will confirm the presence of fluid if the shadow moves (Fig. 83).

Ultrasound
Ultrasound will differentiate fluid from solid pleural lesions and allows guided aspiration of as little as 10 ml loculated fluid.

4.1 Pleural effusion

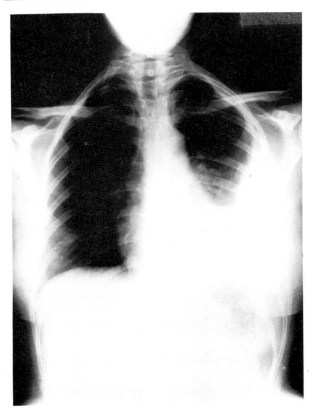

Fig. 80 *Medium-sized left pleural effusion.*

CT scan
A CT scan will differentiate fluid from solid lesions, identify pleural and intrapulmonary lesions and, combined with abdominal scanning, is very useful in the diagnosis of lymphoma in particular.

Management

Pleural aspiration and biopsy
Before therapeutic aspiration is attempted, check that the

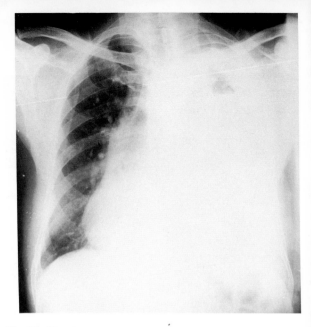

Fig. 81 *Massive left pleural effusion with mediastinal shift.*

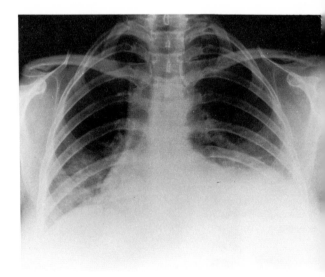

Fig. 82 *Probable bilateral pleural effusions.*

134

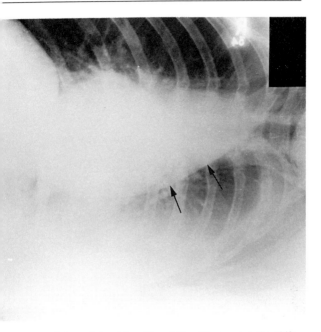

Fig. 83 *Left lateral decubitus film of Fig. 82 showing the shift of fluid with gravity.*

patient does not suffer from hypoproteinaemia, since this may be aggravated by aspiration of further protein. In such cases treatment should be aimed at correcting the hypoproteinaemia; vigorous diuretic therapy may also be necessary, and is also needed for treatment of left ventricular failure. With constrictive pericarditis urgent surgery to relieve the constriction may be necessary (diuretics are contraindicated as the increased filling pressure (preload) is required to maintain the cardiac output).

4.0 Common X-ray presentations

4.1 Pleural effusion

Management of pleural effusions

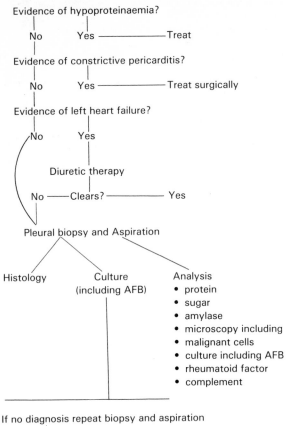

If no diagnosis repeat biopsy and aspiration

If still no diagnosis

Thoracoscopy and biopsy under anaesthesia

4.0 Common X-ray presentations

4.1 Pleural effusion

With all other pleural effusions except in those occurring with an uncomplicated pneumonia, aspiration is usually required, either for diagnostic or therapeutic purposes.

- Confirm the position of the effusion by checking the X-ray (or ultrasound)
- Suppress coughing by giving 10 ml codeine linctus (containing 30 mg codeine phosphate) 30 min before procedure
- Give a premedication of an analgesic such as pethidine together with atropine to prevent pleural shock (vagal reflex)
- Use full sterile conditions
- Select the intercostal space on the patient's back overlying the area of maximum dullness
- Infiltrate down to the pleura with local anaesthetic (1% plain lignocaine) over the upper border of a rib to avoid the neurovascular bundle
- Aspirate the pleural fluid via an aspiration needle, using a syringe and a three-way tap, collecting the fluid in a sterile jug
- It is almost always advisable to perform a pleural biopsy on the first aspiration, having obtained a sample of pleural fluid prior to making the scalpel incision for the Abram's needle (Figs 84 and 85), so that blood is not introduced into the fluid to be analysed. If necessary, the procedure can be repeated after one or two days
- The most important factor in successfully aspirating a chest is to ensure that both the patient and the doctor are comfortably positioned. If the patient becomes uncomfortable for any reason, such as coughing, increasing dyspnoea or pain, the procedure should be discontinued. If aspiration proves unsuccessful because the first attempt was made too close to the diaphragm, a further attempt should be made one rib space higher

Pleural fluid constituents
Having obtained the sample of pleural fluid send it immediately to the laboratory in sterile containers for the following examinations.

Protein estimation. Protein content < 30 g/l = transudate
> 30 g/l = exudate

4.1 Pleural effusion

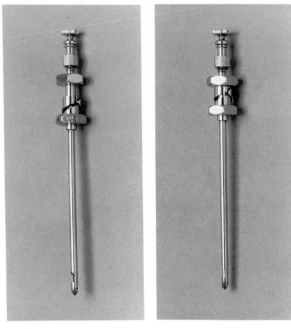

Fig. 84 *(Left) Abram's pleural biopsy needle — open.*

Fig. 85 *(Right) Abram's pleural biopsy needle — closed.*

As mentioned earlier in this chapter this is of considerable diagnostic importance.

Glucose. < 3 mmol/l — occurring with the following complaints:
- rheumatoid arthritis, most commonly
- empyema
- tuberculosis
- many malignant effusions may have low glucose

Amylase. If the level in the pleural fluid is greater than that in the blood — occurs with pancreatitis most commonly

4.0 Common X-ray presentations

4.1 Pleural effusion

Differential cell counts. Lymphocytic effusions simply suggest long-standing effusions — large excesses are suggestive of TB or malignancy.

Polymorphonuclear leucocytic are common and occur with many different aetiologies. Large excess may suggest infection.

Eosinophilic > 10% eosinophils
- idiopathic
- post-traumatic
- hypersensitivity related
- malignant
- pulmonary infarction
- cirrhosis
- sarcoidosis
- rheumatoid

Cytology. Neoplastic cells should be sought as they will be diagnostic for malignancy although often not giving an indication of the primary site of the tumour.

Bacteriology. Routine Gram staining followed by culture may yield common organisms. Tuberculous pleural effusions rarely contain enough organisms to yield a positive direct Ziehl–Neelsen or auramine smear. However, the organism may be seen in the biopsy specimen or be grown from the pleural fluid.

Rheumatoid factor. All rheumatoid effusions have a rheumatoid titre of > 1/160. Rheumatoid factor is also found in low titres in some cases of:
- pneumonia
- malignancy
- TB

Complement. CH_{50} is often undetectable in pleural effusions caused by either SLE or rheumatoid arthritis. $C_4 < 4.5$ mg/l occurs in SLE but not in rheumatoid arthritis or other diseases.

Carcinoembryonic antigen (CEA). Levels > 10 mg/ml are diagnostic of malignancy. However, only 50% of patients with malignancy have elevated levels.

4.0 Common X-ray presentations

4.1 Pleural effusion

Management of special situations

Failure of diagnosis
If a diagnosis is not made after aspiration and biopsy, the procedure should be repeated once. If this still fails to yield the answer, thoracoscopy should be considered unless it is felt there could be a central bronchial carcinoma in which case bronchoscopy is more appropriate. Obviously, both procedures can be performed by a thoracic surgeon under the same anaesthetic.

Recurrent effusions
In patients with malignant or tuberculous effusions, attempts should be made to aspirate to dryness using an intercostal drain. A tuberculous effusion may require several aspirations but will soon respond to chemotherapy.

Repeated aspiration is commonly required in cases of malignant disease, this may be performed regularly on an out-patient basis, so that the patient is away from home for the least time possible. The timing of aspirations will depend on the degree of breathlessness or discomfort. If a thoracic surgeon is available, an abrasive pleurodesis should be considered to obliterate the pleural space, hence providing a more permanent solution. If no surgeon is available, a variety of techniques have been attempted to prevent recurrence, with varying degrees of success. They include the instillation of BCG, thiotepa, nitrogen mustard, mepacrine, radioactive gold, talc, tetracycline, bleomycin or corynebacterium parvum. The secret of success with a pleurodesis is to make sure that all the pleural fluid has been removed through 1 (or 2 intercostal drains) and that the pleural cavity is kept dry by suction if necessary so that the 2 pleural surfaces are in contact with one another.

Complications of pleural effusions and their drainage

- Hydropneumothorax — rarely large, seldom require drainage. Always take chest X-ray after aspiration
- Empyema — detect by presence of pus on aspiration. Treat by adequate drainage through a large intercostal tube and with appropriate systemic antibiotic therapy
- Pleural shock — atropine 0.6 mg i.v. stat.
- Air embolism
- Pulmonary oedema } appropriate resuscitation procedures

4.2 Pneumothorax

Types

Spontaneous pneumothorax
Spontaneous pneumothorax occurs when there is spontaneous escape of air into the pleural space as a result of disease of the visceral pleura, usually through a ruptured pleural bleb or bulla.

Traumatic pneumothorax
Traumatic pneumothorax arises from surgery, stabbings or blunt injuries complicated by fractured ribs.

Tension pneumothorax
Tension pneumothorax develops if air continues to accumulate in the pleural cavity faster than it can be reabsorbed. This accumulation occurs if the ruptured bleb acts as a one-way flap valve. This constitutes an emergency as it is potentially life threatening. It may complicate either a spontaneous or traumatic pneumothorax.

Causes

Common
- Spontaneous rupture of a pleural bleb or bulla. Commoner in young adult males who are often tall and thin. May be recurrent and bilateral; a family history may be found
- Trauma — e.g. surgery, sharp wounds, blunt (non-penetrating compression) injuries, fractured ribs
- Rupture of emphysematous bulla
- Lung biopsies — percutaneous needle or transbronchial — usually small requiring no therapy

Rarer
- Rupture of intrapulmonary cavities into pleural space — staphylococcal abscesses, cavitating carcinoma or tuberculosis
- Iatrogenic factors, e.g. after pleural aspiration, or insertion of subclavian or other central venous catheters
- Resuscitation and ventilation of the newborn, especially the premature or those with respiratory distress
- External cardiac massage and resuscitation in adults
- Positive pressure ventilation

4.2   Pneumothorax

- Asthma
- Cystic fibrosis
- Young adults with rare connective tissue disorders, e.g. Marfan's syndrome or Ehlers-Danlos syndrome

Clinical features

Spontaneous pneumothorax (Fig. 86)
Acute unilateral chest pain will be experienced, which may be associated with breathlessness (depending upon the size of the pneumothorax). Physical signs on the affected side are diminished movement, hyper-resonance, and diminished breath sounds. There may be difficulty in interpreting signs when air

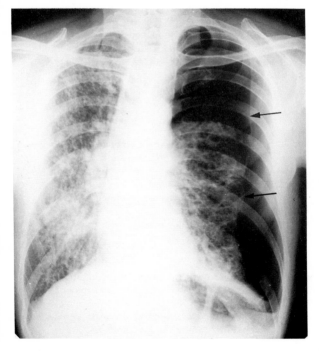

Fig. 86 *Left-side pneumothorax in a patient with extensive bilateral pulmonary fibrosis following a percutaneous drill biopsy.*

4.2 Pneumothorax

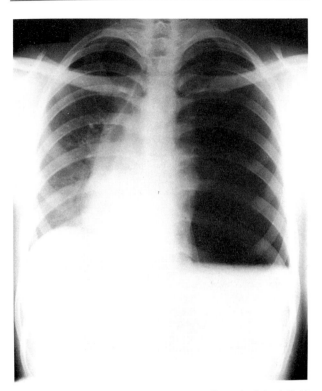

Fig. 87 *Left tension hydropneumothorax. Note the left air fluid level and the absence of lung markings on that side. The heart and trachea are shifted to the right.*

and fluid are simultaneously present (as in a hydropneumothorax). (Hippocratic succussion is the name given to the splashing noise heard if a patient with fluid and air in the pleural cavity moves or is shaken suddenly.)

Tension pneumothorax (Fig. 87)
A tension pneumothorax, recognized by increasing dyspnoea, tachycardia and shift of the trachea and apex beat away from the side of the pneumothorax, requires immediate treatment.

4.0 Common X-ray presentations

4.2 Pneumothorax

Investigations

Chest X-ray is diagnostic — an expiratory film is the best
method of demonstrating a pneumothorax (because it appears
much larger due to the positive intrathoracic pressure tending
to collapse the lung further).

Management

Pain should be controlled with analgesics suited to the severity
of the pain. Small pneumothoraces usually reabsorb
spontaneously. Any pneumothorax which is large enough to
cause distressing dyspnoea, tachycardia, sweating or cyanosis,
must be drained.

Insertion of an intercostal tube
- Drainage is performed under full sterile conditions
- Give the patient a premedication of an analgesic (e.g.
  pethidine) and atropine to avoid 'pleural shock'
- Infiltrate with local anaesthetic, 1% lignocaine over the
  upper edge of a rib in the 4th or 5th intercostal space just
  behind the anterior axillary line. This site is not only more
  comfortable, but also cosmetically more acceptable than
  insertion in the 2nd intercostal space anteriorly
- Use a scalpel to cut a hole through the chest wall large
  enough for the insertion of the intercostal tube. Cut over the
  top edge of a rib to avoid the neurovascular bundle
- Dissect bluntly with scissors or Spencer Wells forceps down
  to the pleura
- Insert the intercostal tube
- Stitch the tube in place. Leave a purse-string suture for when
  the drain is removed.
- Connect it to a bottle containing 500 ml 0.9% saline thereby
  forming an underwater seal
- Keep two clamps by the bed so that the tube can be
  clamped off in emergencies
- Ask the patient to cough to fully reinflate the lung
- Leave the tube in place for 24 hours after it has stopped
  bubbling
- After an X-ray confirming that the lung has reinflated,
  remove the tube
- Close the wound by means of tying the purse-string suture

4.2 Pneumothorax

If the lung fails to reinflate and the tube keeps bubbling, this usually signifies a continuing air leak through the pleura. It is then necessary to apply gentle suction via a Roberts pump to the drainage bottle for several days until the bubbling ceases. Extremely rarely, a thoracotomy is needed to sew up an emphysematous bulla or to divide a pleural adhesion. Occasionally a lung will not re-expand because of mucus plugging in the bronchi — this is easily extracted using a bronchoscope.

Tension pneumothorax
Tension pneumothorax is an acute emergency requiring immediate treatment. If a chest drain is not available, immediately insert the largest available needle through the chest wall into the pneumothorax, thereby relieving the tension and preventing the pneumothorax from increasing in size.

Complications

- Surgical emphysema — skin crepitus due to air leaking along the drainage into subcutaneous tissue — usually requires no therapy. (Exceptionally rarely, however, it may cause either large blood vessel obstruction in the mediastinum impairing venous return to the heart or airway obstruction in the hypopharynx, both of which may be fatal. In these cases, decompression of mediastinal emphysema by cervical skin incisions and tracheostomy can be life-saving)
- Tension pneumothorax — requires immediate drainage
- Haemopneumothorax — requires drainage either via a large basal tube or surgically
- Re-expansion pulmonary oedema — care should be taken to avoid this, since once it has developed there is little specific therapy that can be offered. Many of these patients require artificial ventilation

Prognosis and indications for surgery

About a quarter of all patients with spontaneous pneumothoraces suffer a recurrence of the pneumothorax. With the second occurrence on the same side, consideration should be given to eliminating the pleural space so that no

further pneumothoraces can occur on that side. The 2 methods used are:
- pleurodesis — medical, by putting either sterile talc, kaolin or silver nitrate in the pleural cavity — or surgical, by abrasion
- pleurectomy under general anaesthetic — gives the best long-term results; although it leaves a large scar, to which young women, in particular, often object

Surgical intervention may also be required for:
- simultaneous bilateral pneumothoraces
- haemopneumothorax
- patients whose jobs involve changes in the ambient pressure, such as airline crews and servicemen
- anyone who has had a pneumothorax and who wishes to travel to areas of the globe far from medical centres

Prevention

Although in most patients a pneumothorax is not preventable, special care should be taken with:
- resuscitating the newborn
- positive pressure ventilation, especially with emphysematous patients
- insertion of subclavian or other central venous catheters
- lung biopsies
- chest aspirations
- external cardiac massage

In all these situations it is important to be aware of the possibility of inducing a pneumothorax and to perform a chest X-ray afterwards.

4.3 Mediastinal lesions

Classification

Numerous diseases present with mediastinal lesions which are traditionally subdivided according to their anatomical position as seen on a lateral chest X-ray (Fig. 88).

Superior mediastinum
(manubrium anteriorly, T1–4 posteriorly)

4.0 Common X-ray presentations

4.3 Mediastinal lesions

The following conditions may occur within the superior mediastinum:

• enlarged lymph nodes
  (a) tuberculosis
  (b) sarcoidosis
  (c) lymphoma
  (d) secondaries from a bronchial neoplasm
• retrosternal thyroid
• parathyroid tumours
• thymic tumours
  aortic aneurysm (Fig. 89)
• teratoma
• mediastinal abscess
• oesophageal lesions

Anterior mediastinum

(between body of the sternum and the pericardium, i.e. in front of the heart; Figs 90 and 91)

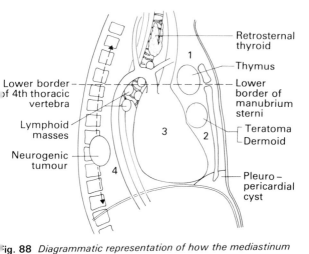

Fig. 88 *Diagrammatic representation of how the mediastinum is divided into four regions to help in the differential diagnosis of masses. 1 Superior mediastinum. 2 Anterior mediastinum. 3 Middle mediastinum. 4 Posterior mediastinum. Also shown are sites of the more common mediastinal tumours, lymph nodes, thyroid and thymus being the most commonly seen.*

4.3 Mediastinal lesions

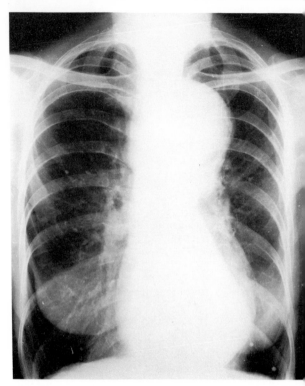

Fig. 89 *Widened superior mediastinum due to an aortic aneurysm.*

The following conditions may occur within the anterior mediastinum:
- thymic tumour or enlargement
- lymphoma
- teratoma
- thyroid
- pleuropericardial (spring water) cyst
- hernia through foramen of Morgagni

Middle mediastinum
(bordered by other 3 regions)

4.3 Mediastinal lesions

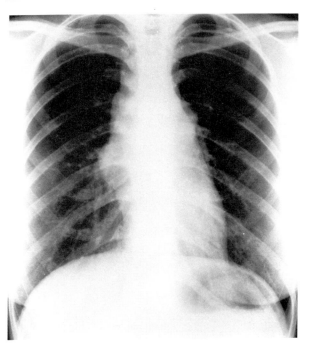

Fig. 90 *PA view of mediastinal mass.*

The following conditions may occur within the middle mediastinum:

- aortic aneurysm
- lymph nodes
  - (a) tuberculosis
  - (b) sarcoidosis
  - (c) lymphoma
  - (d) secondaries from bronchial neoplasm
- lipoma
- bronchogenic cyst

Posterior mediastinum
(pericardium anteriorly, T5–12 posteriorly, i.e. behind the heart; Figs 92–4)

149

4.3 Mediastinal lesions

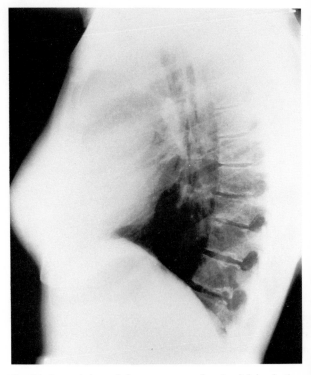

Fig. 91 *Lateral view of the same mass showing it lying in the anterior mediastinum — a thymoma. Note loss of lucency behind the sternum.*

The following conditions may occur within the posterior mediastinum:
- aortic aneurysm
- neurogenic tumours
- oesophageal lesions
- paravertebral abscess
- hernia through foramen of Bochdalek

4.3 Mediastinal lesions

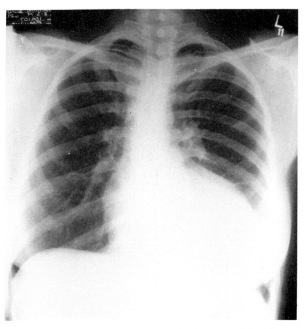

Fig. 92 *Neurogenic posterior mediastinal tumour giving the appearance suggestive of cardiomegaly on the PA film.*

Clinical features

Mediastinal lesions can present in several different ways.

Common presentations
The commonest symptoms or causes of discovering the existence of mediastinal lesions are:

- routine chest X-ray in an asymptomatic patient
- cough and dyspnoea — caused by pressure on the trachea
- dysphagia due to pressure on the oesophagus
- hoarseness if there is a left recurrent laryngeal nerve palsy — this is normally caused by invasion of the nerve by tumour rather than by pressure
- superior vena caval obstruction — local compression
- shortness of breath — phrenic nerve palsy

151

4.3 Mediastinal lesions

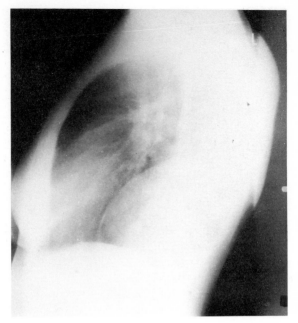

Fig. 93 *Lateral view showing the mass to be lying posteriorly alongside the spine.*

The symptoms which are due to pressure or invasion occur virtually only with malignant tumours or aortic aneurysms. (An exception is bleeding into a retrosternal thyroid, which can cause life-threatening dyspnoea.)

Rarer presentations
Rarer presentations of mediastinal lesions are with:
- thyrotoxicosis — toxic retrosternal goitre
- myasthenia gravis — 20% of patients with myasthenia have a thymoma, some may improve if it is removed
- intercostal and back pain⎫ neurogenic 'dumb-bell'
- spinal cord compression ⎬ tumours in the posterior
⎭ mediastinum

4.3 Mediastinal lesions

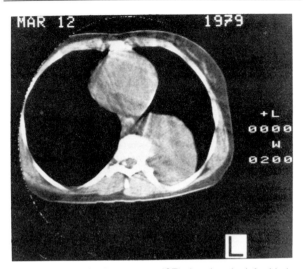

Fig. 94 *Computerized tomogram (CT) showing the left-sided posterior mediastinal mass of neural origin.*

Investigations

- Chest X-ray — PA and lateral
- Fluoroscopic screening to identify vascular structures or check phrenic nerve function
- Tomography or computerized axial tomographic (CAT) scanning
- Barium swallow to check the position of the oesophagus in relation to the mass
- Angiography is useful in outlining aortic aneurysms
- Radioisotope iodine scan sometimes demonstrates a retrosternal thyroid
- Bronchoscopy usually shows only external compression except when there is a primary bronchial carcinoma with secondaries in the mediastinal lymph nodes
- Mediastinoscopy and biopsy are often needed for tissue diagnosis

Management

Surgery
Surgery may be required for the following reasons:
- a diagnostic biopsy
- aortic aneurysms — to prevent rupture
- thymoma — may be malignant and/or cause myasthenia gravis
- thyroid — may haemorrhage and obstruct airway or become toxic
- parathyroid adenoma — hyperparathyroidism
- neurogenic tumours — pain, pressure symptoms, rarely they may be malignant
- teratoma — malignant
- mediastinal abscess — for drainage
- bronchogenic cyst — chronic ill-health akin to bronchiectasis
- dermoid — may become malignant

As many as 20% of 'benign' mediastinal tumours or cysts may become malignant.

Radiotherapy or chemotherapy
Either radiotherapy or chemotherapy or both may be required for the following conditions:
- lymphoma
- metastatic symptoms — bronchial carcinoma being the commonest primary site
- teratoma
- oesophageal cancer

Antibiotics
Antibiotics are used for:
- mediastinal abscess and mediastinitis

Antituberculous chemotherapy
Antituberculous chemotherapy is used with:
- tuberculous lymphadenopathy
- tuberculous paravertebral abscess

Needle aspiration under X-ray guidance
Used for:
- pleuropericardial cyst drainage

4.4   Hilar and mediastinal lymphadenopathy

Causes

The commonest causes of intrathoracic lymphadenopathy are the following:
• tuberculosis (Fig. 95)

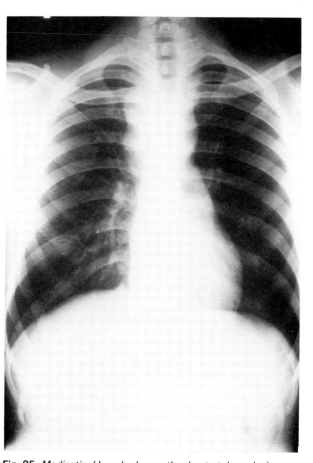

Fig. 95 *Mediastinal lymphadenopathy due to tuberculosis.*

4.4 Hilar and mediastinal lymphadenopathy

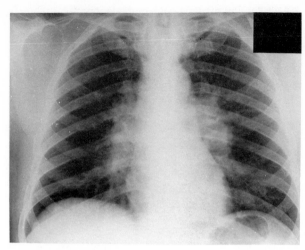

Fig. 96 *Bilateral hilar lymphadenopathy due to sarcoidosis.*

- sarcoidosis (Fig. 96)
- lymphoma (Fig. 97)
- metastatic spread from a bronchial carcinoma

Clinical features

Associated clinical features may be of help in differentiating between these common causes (Table 7).

Tuberculosis
- Often mediastinal or unilateral hilar lymphadenopathy
- The lung fields are usually clear
- Patient is often an immigrant
- The Mantoux or Heaf test is usually strongly positive
- Responds to antituberculous therapy

Sarcoidosis
- Patient often in 3rd or 4th decade
- Frequently a chance finding in an asymptomatic patient
- Common associated symptoms are erythema nodosum (which may also be associated with tuberculosis) and arthralgia

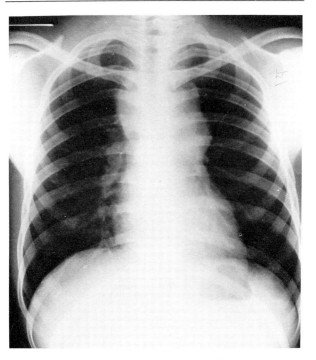

Fig. 97 *Mediastinal mass of glands due to a lymphoma.*

- Usually bilateral hilar lymphadenopathy alone, but may be associated with pulmonary infiltration often in the mid-zones. Mediastinal nodes are often enlarged as well
- Kveim test positive (75%)
- Mantoux test negative (70% at 100 TU)
- Serum angiotensin-converting enzyme often raised
- May show an active alveolitis on bronchoalveolar lavage or gallium scanning
- No response to antituberculous therapy

Lymphoma
- Bilateral or unilateral hilar lymphadenopathy
- Mediastinal involvement can lead to superior vena caval obstruction, phrenic nerve palsy or recurrent laryngeal nerve palsy

157

4.4 Hilar and mediastinal lymphadenopathy

- May be a chance finding or the patient may feel non-specifically unwell
- Fever is common
- Mantoux test usually negative
- The rest of the lung fields are usually clear
- Lymphadenopathy elsewhere and hepatosplenomegaly are commoner than in sarcoidosis (or TB)

Carcinoma of the bronchus
- Unilateral adenopathy, usually with a discernible mass more peripherally on chest X-ray
- Particularly smokers in 5th decade onwards
- SVC obstruction and recurrent laryngeal and phrenic nerve palsies are relatively common
- Finger clubbing may occur

Table 7 Clinical features helpful in the differential diagnosis of hilar lymphadenopathy.

	TB	Sarcoid	Lymphoma	Cancer
Age (yrs)	Any	20–30	20–30	50+
Hilar, one or both	1	Both	Both	1
Mediastinal nodes	+	+	+	+
Response to anti-TB treatment	+	−	−	−
Pressure symptoms, common	−	−	+	+
Fever, common	+	−	+	+
Weight loss	+	±	+	++
Clubbing	−	−	−	+
Lung fields infiltrated	±	+	±	Mass Lesion
Kveim test	−	+ (75%)	−	−
Mantoux test	++	−	+ or −	+ or −
SACE elevated	−	+	−	−
Alveolitis	−	+	−	−

Investigations

After a full history and examination, it is essential to arrive at either a bacteriological or histological diagnosis. The chart

Investigation of intrathoracic lymphadenopathy

Clinical examination
|
Evidence of extrathoracic
lymphadenopathy found

No / Yes

Yes
- hepatomegaly
- palpable lymphaden
  opathy in other
  regions

Biopsy
most accessible
site
|
Diagnosis

No

lung function tests
sputum
  AFB × 3
  cytology × 3
Mantoux test
Kveim test
Angiotensin-converting
  enzyme
Gallium-67 scan

fibreoptic bronchoscopy

Any visible mass?

Yes / No

Yes
Biopsy

No
Transbronchial biopsy + alveolar
lavage even if lung field normal on
CXR

Negative / Positive

Negative
Mediastinoscopy or
mediastinotomy
|
→ Diagnosis ←
- cancer
- TB
- lymphoma
- sarcoid

shows a suggested approach to provide the diagnosis as rapidly as possible.

In areas where tuberculosis is endemic, it may be justifiable to give a trial of antituberculous therapy to patients with lymphadenopathy and a strongly positive Mantoux test and follow the clinical progress, only investigating further those who fail to show response to a month's therapy.

4.5   Solitary lung lesions ('coin' lesions)

Causes

The commonest causes of solitary peripheral lung lesions (Figs 98 and 99) are as follows:
- cancer of the lung (or more rarely a metastasis from cancer elsewhere, e.g. gut, kidney, breast, male and female genitalia or thyroid — these metastases are often multiple)
- tuberculoma
- benign tumour
- pneumonia (especially lipoid)
- abscess
- infarcted lung
- encysted pleural effusion

Regrettably, malignancy is by far the most common cause of solitary lung lesions in the UK. Rarer causes include:
- hydatid cyst
- rheumatoid nodule
- histoplasmosis

Investigations

When a solitary lung lesion is identified, it is very important:
1. to try and discover how long it has been there
2. to discover if it has altered in size. Thus during a full clinical examination it is essential to discover whether the patient has ever had a previous chest X-ray (e.g. mass X-ray, routine pre-employment, preoperative). If so, it is essential to obtain the films for comparison. Mass X-rays are usually retained for 5 years, occasionally for 7 years. If the lesion

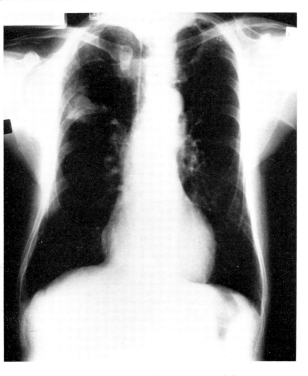

Fig. 98 *Solitary 'coin' lesion in the right upper lobe.*

has been present for several years, and is unchanged in
size, there is no real need to investigate further at this
stage.

If there are no old films or if the lesion is proved to be of recent
origin, the main anxiety is that of there being a bronchial
carcinoma. Sputum examination for cytology and AFB and
fibreoptic bronchoscopy with biopsy and/or brushing of any
visible lesion, are all required. If bronchoscopy is negative, then
a percutaneous needle biopsy of the mass should be performed
under X-ray control (if it is in a safe position).

If other widespread lesions are seen on tomography or CT

4.5 Solitary lung lesions ('coin' lesions)

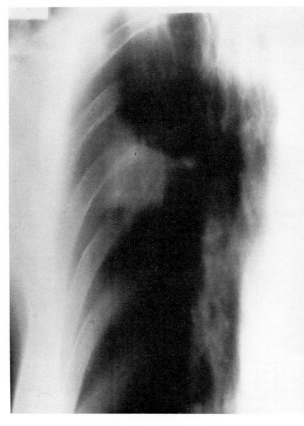

Fig. 99 *Tomogram of the solitary lesion in Fig. 98 showing that there is neither calcification nor cavitation.*

scan, the likelihood of multiple metastases rises. Calcification of the lesion suggests tuberculosis or, more rarely, a hamartoma.

The tuberculin test is only helpful if negative; a tuberculoma is then unlikely. If the history, place of domicile and travel indicate it, histoplasmin skin test, hydatid and histoplasma CFTs may be useful.

Investigation of solitary lung lesions

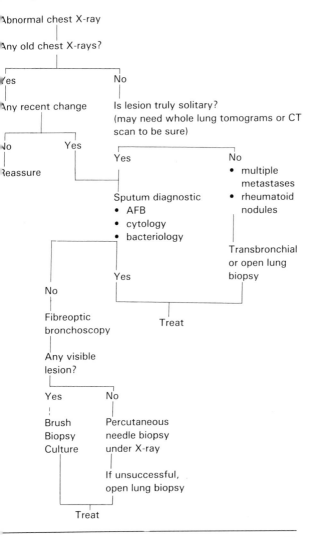

Abnormal chest X-ray
|
Any old chest X-rays?

Yes — No

Yes branch:
Any recent change

No — Yes

No → Reassure

No branch:
Is lesion truly solitary?
(may need whole lung tomograms or CT scan to be sure)

Yes — No

No:
- multiple metastases
- rheumatoid nodules

Transbronchial or open lung biopsy

Yes:
Sputum diagnostic
- AFB
- cytology
- bacteriology

Yes → Treat

No →
Fibreoptic bronchoscopy

Any visible lesion?

Yes — No

Yes:
Brush
Biopsy
Culture

No:
Percutaneous needle biopsy under X-ray

If unsuccessful, open lung biopsy

Treat

4.5 Solitary lung lesions ('coin' lesions)

Thoracotomy and resection may be needed for diagnosis if other investigations have failed.

Management

Treatment is directed to the specific cause (see individual diseases). However, if the histology is one of an adenocarcinoma, it is difficult to be certain that the lung lesion is the primary. If the neoplastic lesions are multiple (Fig. 100), clearly they are secondaries. The question then often arises as to how far one should search for a primary lesion.

In many cases, finding the primary will neither help the patient nor alter therapy. However, in the case of certain primary lesions, chemotherapy may help, e.g. when located in:

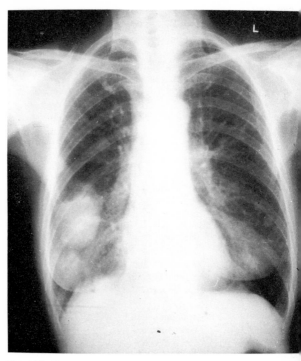

Fig. 100 *Two 'cannonball' metastases in the right lower lobe.*

4.0 Common X-ray presentations

4.5 Solitary lung lesions ('coin' lesions)

- thyroid
- prostate
- breast
- kidney
- testis

Some renal secondaries may regress after resection of the primary. A large bowel primary is worth discovering, so that palliative surgery can be performed to avoid large bowel obstruction. However, it is unjustifiable to perform a routine barium meal and enema and intravenous pyelogram on all patients who have multiple metastases and who do not have symptoms relating to the particular system. In a fit, young patient a solitary lung secondary may be worth resecting in addition to the primary, but one should make certain by CT scan that it is indeed a solitary secondary.

4.6 Lung cavities and abscesses (Figs 101 and 102)

Causes

Emphysematous bullae are usually not difficult to diagnose when seen on X-ray. It is more difficult to diagnose the exact aetiology of a cavitating pneumonia or thick-walled cavities. The features of the most common causes of such cavitation are shown in the following table.

Table 8 Common causes of cavitation.

Cause	Distribution	Frequently multiple	Usual age
Tuberculosis	Upper lobe	Yes	Any
Carcinoma of the bronchus	Anywhere	No	45+
Klebsiella pneumonia	Upper lobe	Yes	60+
Staphylococcal pneumonia	Anywhere	Yes	20–30 or 60+
Lung abscess	Anywhere	No	Any

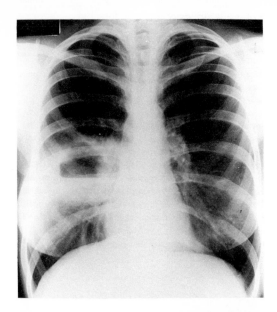

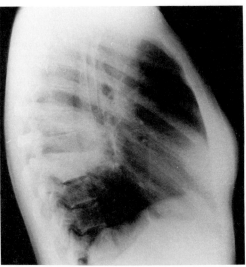

Fig. 101 *(a, top) and (b, bottom) Lung abscess in the apex of the right lower lobe. Note the air fluid level in the cavity.*

4.0 Common X-ray presentations

4.6 Lung cavities and abscesses

Lung abscesses are often caused either by bronchial
obstruction with:
• carcinoma
• foreign bodies

or by impaired tracheobronchial clearance such as occurs with:
• aspiration
• coma
• alcoholics
• bronchiectasis
• laryngeal incompetence
• oesophageal lesions

Rare causes of cavitation
• Pulmonary infarct
• Emboli from right-sided endocarditis
• Progressive massive fibrosis
• Caplan's syndrome
• Hydatid disease
• Nocardiasis
• Histoplasmosis
• Coccidioidomycosis
• Blastomycosis
• Actinomycosis

Investigations

A full history is essential. The doctor should enquire particularly
for contact with tuberculosis, smoking, foreign travel, recent
influenza.

Blood count
Neutrophilia in bacterial infection.

Sputum
• Gram stain — culture and sensitivity
• Cytology for malignant cells × 3
• Stain for AFB × 3

Blood culture
On 3 occasions in febrile patients.

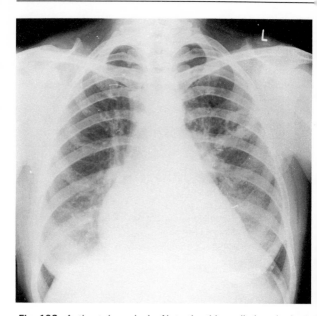

Fig. 102 *Active tuberculosis. Note the thin-walled cavity in the left upper lobe.*

Bronchoscopy
The bronchial washings and aspirate are examined and cultured for bacteria, especially if there is no sputum. Bronchoscopy is also required to exclude the presence of a foreign body or neoplasm.

Percutaneous needle biopsy
This is performed under X-ray control in afebrile patients with solitary lesions in whom a cancer is likely. Similarly, large abscesses can be drained and antibiotics instilled into the cavity.

Complement fixation tests
This is used for the rarer infectious diseases in difficult cases.

Barium swallow
Barium swallow will reveal if there is any continuing aspiration.

4.6 Lung cavities and abscesses

Therapy

This is directed at the underlying cause:

- i.v. penicillin G *and* flucloxacillin for staphylococcal pneumonia
- rifampicin, isoniazid and ethambutol for tuberculosis
- cotrimoxazole or ampicillin and gentamicin for Klebsiella
- surgery, radiotherapy or chemotherapy for cancer
- drainage for abscess
- removal of foreign bodies

4.7 Diffuse lung shadowing

Causes

A common diagnostic problem met in hospital practice is the interpretation of a diffusely abnormal chest X-ray, both lung fields having nodular, reticular or diffusely abnormal shadowing.

The asymptomatic patient
The likely causes are:

- sarcoidosis — hilar adenopathy may also be present
- pneumoconiosis — occupational history will often give the diagnosis
- 'burnt out' fibrosing alveolitis

Clinical presentation is usually by a mass miniature X-ray or a pre-employment X-ray. Patients with marked changes through diseases other than these are usually symptomatic or febrile and acutely unwell.

The symptomatic patient, afebrile and not acutely ill
The common presenting symptoms are progressive breathlessness coupled with a persistent dry cough. Weight loss and malaise are common and haemoptysis is also sometimes found.

With this presentation the differential diagnosis is:

- diffuse malignant metastases and/or lymphangitis carcinomatosis from 1 of the following organs:
  (i) bronchus

4.7 Diffuse lung shadowing

   (ii)   gastrointestinal tract
   (iii) breast
   (iv) kidney
   (v)   thyroid
   (vi) prostate
   (vii) testis
- tuberculosis
- sarcoidosis
- cryptogenic fibrosing alveolitis
- extrinsic allergic alveolitis
- rheumatoid lung
- lymphoma
- asbestosis
- histoplasmosis ⎫
- blastomycosis ⎬ in the relevant geographical areas
- coccidioidomycosis ⎭

The symptomatic patient, febrile and acutely ill
In these patients the main differential diagnosis lies between:
- tuberculosis
- bronchopneumonia
- viral or atypical pneumonia
- extrinsic allergic alveolitis
- histoplasmosis ⎫
- coccidioidomycosis ⎬ in the relevant geographical areas
- blastomycosis ⎭
- pneumocystis pneumonia — especially in the immunosuppressed

Clinical features

In addition to the usual full systematic questioning, patients should be asked particularly about the following:
- occupation — especially farming, coal mining and asbestos exposure
- contact with infectious diseases, especially tuberculosis
- pets and hobbies (e.g. racing pigeons)
- foreign travel
- previous surgery and medical treatment, particularly for malignant disease, e.g. mastectomy
- previous diseases
- possible antigen exposure, if history suggests allergic

170

4.7 Diffuse lung shadowing

alveolitis
- drug therapy

Examination will show whether the patient is febrile and acutely unwell or not. Most of the diseases are associated with restricted chest movements and bilateral crepitations. Finger clubbing is found commonly in lung cancer, fibrosing alveolitis and asbestosis but not in the other diseases. In most patients, further investigations will be needed.

Investigations

The following investigations will lead to a specific diagnosis in the majority of cases.

Sputum
- Gram stain — culture and sensitivity
- Auramine or Z–N stain for tubercle bacilli × 3
- Cytology for malignant cells × 3

Blood cultures
Blood cultures may yield a bacterial pathogen in pneumonia.

Tuberculin skin test
Mantoux, Heaf or Tine tests are usually strongly positive in tuberculosis, but can be negative in the very severely ill patient with tuberculosis. Tuberculin tests are usually negative in sarcoidosis, tuberculin sensitivity may also be lost in lymphoma and carcinoma.

Kveim skin test
If a Kveim skin test is positive, it is virtually diagnostic for sarcoidosis.

Angiotensin-converting enzyme
This is elevated in sarcoidosis.

Serum precipitins
Serum precipitins to aspergillus, mouldy hay, pigeon or bird proteins are caused by the relevant antigen in extrinsic allergic alveolitis.

Rheumatoid factor
This is found in rheumatoid arthritis and fibrosing alveolitis.

4.7 Diffuse lung shadowing

Antinuclear factor
This is found in fibrosing alveolitis and SLE.

Cold agglutinins
Cold agglutinins are often present in mycoplasma infection.

Mycoplasma complement fixation test

Histoplasmin test (in USA)

Coccidioidin test (in USA)

Lung function tests
A restrictive defect with impaired gas transfer is present in the majority of symptomatic patients.

Lung biopsies
Despite the above investigations, a tissue diagnosis is usually needed, first by means of a transbronchial biopsy. If this is non-diagnostic, then open lung biopsy is needed.

Special diagnostic problems

Three special situations may occur.
1. An acutely ill patient with no diagnosis, but diffuse shadowing on chest X-ray. In these circumstances it is best to start treatment whilst awaiting the results of cultures and transbronchial lung biopsy. One needs to cover for miliary tuberculosis (rifampicin, isoniazid and ethambutol) and bronchopneumonia (ampicillin and gentamicin). If there is any suspicion of mycoplasma, it is best to include erythromycin or tetracycline. Many of these drugs can be stopped after 24 hours when cultures become available or as the patient is seen to recover and the X-ray clears (days/weeks in pneumonia, weeks/months in miliary TB).
2. The patient who is too old or unfit for an open lung biopsy and who has had a non-contributory transbronchial biopsy. The diagnosis usually lies between sarcoidosis, tuberculosis, fibrosing alveolitis or malignant metastases. Give a trial of antituberculous chemotherapy for 2–3 months and judge response whilst awaiting the results of the Kveim test. If there is no response, then try steroid therapy (30 mg daily) — sarcoidosis and sometimes fibrosing alveolitis will

respond. If the patient deteriorates continuously, malignancy is then most likely. It should be emphasized that with the ease and acceptability of transbronchial biopsies (repeated if necessary) this situation is now much less common than it was at one time and it is now nearly always possible to arrive at a diagnosis.

A more common problem nowadays is the following:
3. Multiple metastases 'hunting the primary'. The primary may be obvious from the history, e.g. previous mastectomy. Primary sites should be divided into those which are worth detecting because curative therapy may be offered, and those primaries about which one can do little and therefore an extensive search is not warranted. With an adenocarcinoma secondary in the lung, there is only a 30% success rate of finding a primary even at post-mortem — this underlines the futility of the exercise in most patients.

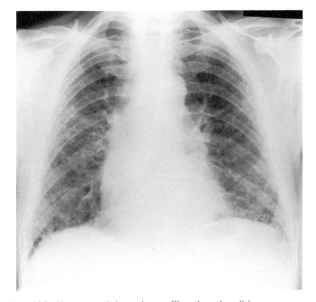

Fig. 103 *Honeycomb lung due to fibrosing alveolitis.*

4.8   Honeycomb lung (Fig. 103)

Causes

Honeycombing is the presence of either localized or diffuse thick-walled cysts, varying from 0.5–2.0 cm in size, which do not fill on bronchograms. Bronchiectasis can produce a very similar plain X-ray, but of course the abnormal shadows fill on bronchography.

Localized form of a disease
- Sarcoidosis
- Asbestosis
- Tuberculosis
- Systemic sclerosis
- Berylliosis
- Rheumatoid lung

Diffuse bilateral disease — 'honeycomb' lung
- Diffuse fibrosing alveolitis
- Histiocytosis X (eosinophilic granuloma, Letterer-Siwe, Hand-Schüller-Christian disease)
- Tuberculosis
- Neurofibromatosis

5.0 Some important diseases

5.0 Some important diseases

5.0 Some important diseases

5.1 Upper respiratory tract infections

This extremely common group of conditions account for about 50% of the work lost in the UK each year. The vast majority are caused by viruses. They can be divided into a number of types according to the main symptoms.

The common cold

Common colds are caused by rhinovirus, parainfluenza, echovirus, coxsackie or respiratory syncytial viruses. Symptoms include runny nose, sneezing, watering eyes, headache and malaise.

Sore throats

Common viral causes include adenovirus, parainfluenza, echovirus and coxsackie. The commonest bacterial cause is the haemolytic streptococcus. The main symptom is pharyngitis, often with hoarseness, malaise and fever. Infectious mononucleosis should also be remembered as a cause of sore throats — lymphadenopathy is always present.

Influenza

Caused by influenza A, B and C viruses. Symptoms include fever, prostration, malaise, myalgia, headaches, cough, sore throat and tracheitis. Rarely in young adults and the elderly is it complicated by staphylococcal pneumonia.

Influenza vaccination
Although specific immunization against influenza is effective (70% protection) in studies on volunteers, there has been little success in controlling epidemics. There are 3 problems. The first is in raising a vaccine to the specific circulating viruses whose antigens are changing rapidly. Currently, two subtypes of influenza A, HINI and H3N2, are circulating and undergoing antigenic shift independently. The second is in formulating a vaccine according to the host defences of the population. Finally, there is the timing of the vaccination; the spread of the disease may be too rapid to develop a specific vaccine and the

5.0 Some important diseases

5.1 Upper respiratory tract infections

immunity is short-lived (6 months) because of the character of antihaemagglutinin antibodies.

As yet, there is no evidence to support the practice of giving the present commercially available vaccine to patients with chronic respiratory disease each winter.

Croup

Croup usually occurs in young children. Viral causes include respiratory syncytial virus, parainfluenza adenovirus and influenza viruses. The main bacterial cause is *Haemophilus influenzae*. Symptoms are cough and shortness of breath. Stridor is caused by laryngeal oedema.

Therapy

Upper respiratory tract infections, with the exception of croup and streptococcal sore throats, do not require specific therapy, although secondary bacterial infection complicating influenza will require antibiotics. Croup therapy includes:
- steam inhalations
- oxygen — 35%
- broad-spectrum antibiotics — (ampicillin)
- bronchodilators — (salbutamol via nebuliser)
- steroids in severe cases

Streptococcal sore throat requires penicillin V 250 mg 6-hourly for 10 days (erythromycin if allergic to penicillin).

5.2 Acute tracheitis and bronchitis

Causes

Acute lower respiratory tract infection in previously healthy adults is usually associated with a viral upper respiratory tract infection — a cold or 'flu. In chronic bronchitis, acute bacterial exacerbations due to *Haemophilus influenzae* or *Streptococcus pneumoniae* are common.

5.0 Some important diseases

5.2 Acute tracheitis and bronchitis

Clinical features

Common
- Fever
- Cough
- Purulent sputum
- Retrosternal soreness
- Wheeze

Rarer
- Breathlessness
- Haemoptysis

Investigations

The following investigations and results are found with these conditions:
- white cell count elevated
- Gram stain and culture of sputum yield pathogen
- chest X-ray normal
- peak flow rate ⎫ abnormal only when there is
- blood gases ⎭ co-existent chronic bronchitis or asthma

Therapy

Cough suppressant
Codeine linctus 10 ml p.r.n.

Antibiotics
If there is proven bacterial infection, give broad-spectrum antibiotics such as:
- amoxycilin 250 mg 8-hourly

or:
- cotrimoxazole 960 mg 12-hourly

or:
- oxytetracycline 250 mg 6-hourly

Bronchodilators
Terbutaline 500 μg or fenoterol 360 μg or salbutamol 200 μg 6-hourly (via metered dose aerosol) for wheeze and airways obstruction.

5.0 Some important diseases

5.2 Acute tracheitis and bronchitis

Physiotherapy
Physiotherapy is important to aid expectoration of sputum.

Oxygen (if there is hypoxia)

5.3 Pneumonia

Causes

Pneumonia means infection of the lung parenchyma (acinus). It may be classified according to the causes.

Bacterial infections
- *Streptococcus pneumoniae* — the pneumococcus
- *Haemophilus influenzae*
- *Staphylococcus aureus*
- *Klebsiella pneumoniae*
- *Mycobacterium tuberculosis*
- *Pseudomonas pyocyanea*

Mycoplasma and Q fever (Coxiella burneti)

Legionnaire's disease
- *Legionella pneumophila*

Ornithosis
- *Chlamydia psittaci*

Viral infections
- Adenovirus
- Respiratory syncytial virus
- Influenza
- Coxsackie
- Enteric cytopathic human orphan (ECHO) virus
- Ebstein-Barr (EB) virus
- Varicella zoster
- Cytomegalovirus

Fungal infections
- Aspergillus
- Histoplasmosis
- Coccidioidomycosis

5.3 Pneumonia

- Blastomycosis
- Nocardia
- Candida

Protozoa
- Toxoplasmosis
- *Pneumocystis carinii*

Aspiration

Radiation
An alternative way of classifying pneumonia is by the anatomical distribution, i.e. lobar pneumonia, for example, due to the pneumococcus; or bronchopneumonia, for example, due to *H. influenzae*. Classification by cause is more helpful because it aids in the choice of specific antimicrobial therapy.

Clinical features — general

Groups at risk
Although most cases of pneumonia occur sporadically there are certain groups of people or patients who are at greater risk:
- those in close communities or institutions — hospitals, schools, barracks, prisons, hostels
- chronic bronchitics or bronchiectatics
- patients with any other chronic lung disease
- the immunosuppressed, particularly the very old or very young or patients with cancer, leukaemia or acquired immunodeficiency syndrome (AIDS)
- patients with cirrhosis and renal failure
- postsplenectomy or hyposplenism
- postviral infection
- prolonged bed rest (cerebrovascular accident, trauma, intensive care)
- pulmonary oedema
- aspiration of food
- alcoholics and other drug addicts
- patients on steroid or cytotoxic therapy

Symptoms
These may include:
- malaise and prostration following an upper respiratory tract infection

181

5.3 Pneumonia

- fever and sweating
- cough
- purulent sputum, sometimes with blood
- pleurisy

Signs
These may include:
- fever
- tachypnoea
- confusion
- cyanosis
- herpes labialis (with pneumococcus)
- diminished movement ⎫
- dull percussion note ⎪ Over the affected areas: often
- crepitations ⎬ the crepitations are the only
- bronchial breathing ⎪ abnormal chest sign — particularly
- pleural rub ⎭ in the early stages

Investigations

Chest X-ray
PA and lateral views show areas of consolidation with, on occasions, air bronchograms. The distribution is lobular or lobar with the pneumococcus. It is patchy or diffuse with other causes. Other complications which may be seen are abscesses, collapse (with mucus plugs) and small pleural effusions.

Blood count
An elevated white count (neutrophilia) is found in bacterial infections. Cold agglutinins occur with mycoplasma infection.

Sputum
- Gram stain and culture for bacteria and fungi
- Auramine (or Z–N) stain for mycobacterium tuberculosis
- Culture of sputum and nasal washings for viruses

Blood culture
Often positive in pneumococcal pneumonia.

Serology
Paired acute and convalescent samples will provide a retrospective diagnosis of viral and mycoplasma pneumonias; a fourfold rise in titre being diagnostic. Legionnaire's disease is

confirmed by an indirect fluorescent antibody test. Precipitins to aspergillus are worth performing in the immunosuppressed patient at risk from a fungal pneumonia.

Alveolar lavage and transbronchial lung biopsy
Alveolar lavage together with histology and culture may be useful in diagnosis of 'obscure' pneumonias such as the pneumonias due to *Pneumocystis carinii* and aspergillus occurring in the immunosuppressed.

Blood gases
Hypoxia with a normal or low $Paco_2$ is the usual pattern because of the V/Q mismatch. Elevation of $Paco_2$ occurs with co-existent severe airways obstruction or ventilatory failure.

Complications

Relatively common
- Pleural effusion or empyema
- Lung abscess
- Respiratory failure — type 1
- Bacteraemia
- Cor pulmonale (with chronic bronchitis or other severe pre-existing lung disease)

Rarer
- Pericarditis
- Myocarditis
- Cholestatic jaundice
- Meningitis (pneumococcus)

Differential diagnosis

Once the patient has been examined and a chest X-ray has been taken, pulmonary embolism and tuberculosis are the only common diagnoses which, in practice, can prove difficult to differentiate from an established pneumonia. However, frank haemoptysis is rare in pneumonia and purulent sputum is unusual in the initial stage of pulmonary embolism. Sources for pulmonary embolism (deep vein thromboses, DVTs) should be sought. Pulmonary tuberculosis may be confused with pneumonia even with the help of a chest X-ray; hence the

importance of examining every patient's sputum for
mycobacteria on at least three occasions.

Clinical features of specific pneumonias

Pneumococcal
This was one of the most feared diseases in pre-antibiotic days,
killing numerous young adults. The terms double or single
pneumonia, still heard, refer to the number of lobes affected.
Outbreaks often occur in institutions. The patient may be
almost unaffected by the disease or virtually moribund. Herpes
labialis is frequently seen. The typical pneumonic distribution is
lobar with signs of consolidation. The sputum is typically
'rusty'. Pleurisy with a pleural rub is common, often followed
by a pleural effusion. Other complications include septicaemia,
meningitis, endocarditis, pericarditis, myocarditis, peritonitis,
empyema and cholestatic jaundice.

Staphylococcal
Although pneumonia during or following influenza is rare, when
it occurs the commonest pathogen is *Staph. aureus*. It is also a
common pathogen in young children, the elderly and
hospitalized patients. Another special group at risk are drug
addicts who may have a right-sided staphylococcal
endocarditis with embolic pneumonia. Staphylococcal
pneumonia is often a bilateral cavitating bronchopneumonia
(Fig. 104).

Klebsiella
Klebsiella is a serious pathogen in the elderly, causing
cavitation with expansion, particularly in the upper lobes, but
other lobes are also commonly affected.

Pseudomonas
This is a common pathogen in bronchiectasis and cystic
fibrosis. Otherwise it occurs mainly in hospitals, particularly in
intensive care units and after surgery. The patients have often
either had numerous antibiotics or had airways surgery or,
endotracheal intubation. Pseudomonas may occur in the
sputum as a commensal; thus, with no other evidence of
pneumonia, treatment is unnecessary.

5.3 Pneumonia

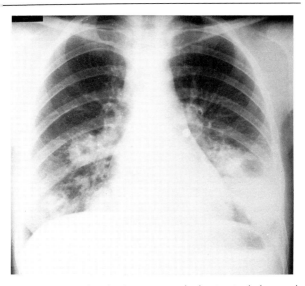

Fig. 104 *Bilateral cavitating pneumonia due to staphylococcal pneumonia. Note the air fluid levels in the cavities.*

Primary atypical pneumonia (mycoplasma)

Primary atypical pneumonia occurs in closed communities; some of the largest outbreaks have been in army recruits. The disease often presents insidiously as a prolonged pneumonia which fails to clear with 2–3 weeks treatment using conventional broad-spectrum antibiotics. Particular features include flu-like symptoms of headaches and myalgia. Chest X-ray shows consolidation with no characteristic diagnostic features. A very high ESR with cold agglutinins are supportive evidence for the diagnosis, which is confirmed by a fourfold rise in antibody titres over 10–14 days. High antibody titres may persist for several years, therefore a single high titre is unhelpful.

Psittacosis (ornithosis)

Chlamydia psittaci is an intracellular organism which causes a severe interstitial pneumonia. Cardiac valvular involvement may occur. The infection may be contracted from contact with sick birds — classically parrots — but other animals may also be vectors. A fourfold rise in antibody titre over 10 days or cell culture of the organism from blood or sputum is needed to confirm the diagnosis.

Virus pneumonia
No specific therapy is available and it is rare to make a diagnosis other than in retrospect from rises in viral antibody titres. Clinically, the disease is associated with typical 'viral' symptoms — fever, headache and myalgia.

Legionnaire's disease (pneumophila legionella)
Outbreaks of Legionnaire's disease occur particularly in hotels and hospitals, often connected with contaminated water and air conditioning. Legionnaire's disease is more common than was first realized. The mortality rate is probably less than 10% In addition to the usual pneumonic features, the particular features suggesting Legionnaire's disease include some of the following:
- gastrointestinal upset
- confusion, encephalopathy
- hyponatraemia
- lymphopenia
- hepatitis
- haematuria

Pneumocystis carinii
A rare infection in adults, *Pneumocystis carinii* is almost invariably found in the immunosuppressed especially in AIDS. The usual signs and symptoms are:
- dry cough
- breathlessness
- fever
- cyanosis
- crepitations bilaterally

Alveolar lavage or lung biopsy are necessary for diagnosis.

Other diseases with associated pneumonia
Other rare diseases with associated pneumonia or common diseases in which pneumonia is a rare complication are:
- toxoplasmosis
- measles
- whooping cough
- chickenpox

- brucellosis
- anthrax
- nocardia
- actinomycosis
- plague

Histoplasmosis and coccidioidomycosis

Both histoplasmosis and coccidioidomycosis are very rare in the UK, but are common in parts of the USA. Both occur either as a primary disease, during which the patient is usually well, or as a chronic granulomatous form similar to post primary adult tuberculosis, in which the patient is sick with a chronic pneumonic illness.

Therapy

Analgesia for pleuritic pain

Effective pain relief is essential to aid deep respiration, effective coughing and physiotherapy. Treatment varies according to the degree of pain, as follows:

- mild pain — soluble aspirin 600 mg 4-hourly, or paracetamol 1 g 4-hourly, in patients who are sensitive to aspirin
- moderate pain — dihydrocodeine 30 mg or pentazocine 50 mg orally 4-hourly
- severe pain — pethidine 100 mg i.m., or morphine 10 mg i.m.

Such opiates depress respiratory drive and should be avoided in patients with associated chronic bronchitis or any other patient with an elevated Pa_{CO_2}.

Oxygen

Initially, administration of oxygen is 35% by ventimask (unless the patient has an elevated Pa_{CO_2}, when 24% should be given). Higher concentrations can be given if 35% does not provide adequate oxygenation.

Physiotherapy

Percussion and postural drainage should be instituted ideally 15–20 minutes after the dose of analgesia. In acute pneumonia physiotherapy should be performed 6-hourly.

5.0 Some important diseases

5.3 Pneumonia

Hydration

In severely ill patients, fluid balance must be carefully controlled; this is particularly true in Legionnaire's disease. A central venous pressure line is useful to avoid over-hydration, to administer antibiotics, and for parenteral nutrition if required.

Antibiotics

These are the mainstay of treatment of bacterial pneumonia. There are 6 groups of anti-bacterial drugs. The first 4 are bactericidal, the last 2 are largely bacteriostatic.

1. Interference with the bacterial cell wall — penicillin and cephalosporins.
2. Disruption of cell membrane — nystatin, amphotericin.
3. Interference with RNA polymerase — rifampicin.
4. Degradation of DNA — metronidazole.
5. Interference with folate manufacture — sulphonamides and trimethoprim.
6. Interference with protein synthesis on the ribosomes — (a) streptomycin, gentamicin (both bactericidal); (b) erythromycin, tetracycline, chloramphenicol, clindomycin (all bacteriostatic)

Initial antibiotic choice is shown in Table 9. Within 24–48 hours, culture and sensitivity of organisms will be available, the likely sensitivities include:

Pneumococcus	— penicillin or erythromycin
H. influenzae	— ampicillin or amoxycillin; or cotrimoxazole; or oxytetracycline
Staph. aureus	— flucloxacillin
Klebsiella	— cotrimoxazole; or gentamicin; or tobramycin
Pseudomonas	— piperacillin or azlocillin
Mycoplasma	— oxytetracycline or erythromycin
Legionnaire's disease	— erythromycin or rifampicin
Psittacosis	— oxytetracycline
Pneumocystis	— cotrimoxazole in high dose (3.84 g 12-hourly)

Prognosis

The outlook of an uncomplicated pneumonia in previously fit adults is good with correct therapy. Where pneumonia

Table 9 Initial antibiotic therapy in pneumonia.

| | Gram stain result | | | |
Negative	Gram-positive	Gram-negative	Gram-negative in chronic bronchitis	Fungal
Moderately ill	*Pneumococcus* Benzylpenicillin i.v. 2 megaunits 12-hourly until patient is significantly better, then Penicillin V 500 mg 6-hourly orally for 7 days	Ampicillin 500 mg 6-hourly orally and Gentamicin 80 mg (1.5 mg/kg) i.v. or i.m. 8-hourly (check renal function and gentamicin levels)	Ampicillin 500 mg 6-hourly orally for 10 days as *H. influenzae* most likely organism	If renal function normal, amphotericin 250 μg/kg daily, increasing to 1 mg/kg daily if tolerated. Total dose 2–4 g or ketoconazole 200 mg 12-hourly orally
Ampicillin 500 mg 6-hourly orally for 10 days	*Staphylococcus aureus* Flucloxacillin 500 mg 6-hourly i.v. until patient is significantly better, then orally for 10 days			
Very ill Ampicillin 1 g 6-hourly i.v. and gentamicin 80 mg (1.5 mg/kg) i.v. 8-hourly (check renal function and gentamicin levels)				

complicates other diseases or occurs in neonates, the elderly or
in those otherwise immunosuppressed, the prognosis is much
poorer. Fungal and pneumocystis pneumonia have particularly
poor prognoses.

5.4 Bronchiectasis

Bronchiectasis is the persistent dilation of bronchi and
bronchioles. It can be either saccular (cystic) or cylindrical.
Bronchiectasis is the result of severe or persistent lower
respiratory tract infection. It now occurs more rarely, possibly
because of the more liberal use of antibiotics in childhood.

Causes

- Severe lung infection in childhood, e.g. measles, whooping
  cough or bronchiolitis
- Tuberculosis
- Allergic aspergillosis — associated with mucus plugging and
  asthma
- Hypogammaglobulinaemia — congenital or acquired IgA
  deficiency
- Chronic sinusitis
- Kartagener's syndrome (situs inversus, chronic sinusitis,
  bronchiectasis) and the immotile cilia syndrome
- Sequestrated segment (non-functioning lung with blood
  supply directly from the aorta rather than from the
  pulmonary artery)
- Bronchial obstruction due to foreign body or adenoma
- Rheumatoid arthritis or ulcerative colitis (both rare causes)

Clinical features

Common symptoms
- Persistent cough
- Copious purulent sputum
- Intermittent haemoptysis

Common signs
- Halitosis
- Coarse crackles over affected area

5.0 Some important diseases

5.4 Bronchiectasis

- Finger clubbing (30%)
- Wheezes with associated chronic bronchitis, asthma or bronchopulmonary aspergillosis

Complications

Common
- Recurrent infectious episodes
- Pneumonia

Rare
- Amyloidosis
- Brain abscess

Investigations

Sputum
Bacterial culture of sputum often yields *Haemophilus influenzae*,
Strep. pneumoniae, staphylococci or anaerobes. *Aspergillus fumigatus* may be identified.

Skin tests for aspergillus

Aspergillus serum precipitins

} to diagnose aspergillosis

Serum immunoglobulins
Check for hypogammaglobulinaemia.

Chest X-ray
This is often normal, however, streaky shadows 'tramlines' or ring shadows may be seen on the PA or lateral.

Respiratory function
Spirometry often shows an obstructive picture. The amount of reversibility to β agonists should be assessed.

Bronchoscopy
This is mainly useful in locating the site of any bleeding and to exclude an adenoma or foreign body.

Bronchogram
Although a clinical diagnosis is often obvious, a definitive

diagnosis can only be made by performing a bronchogram. This should only be performed:
- if the knowledge is going to help in the management (e.g. locating a lobe which could be resected)
- when respiratory function is optimal after postural drainage, physiotherapy and bronchodilators
- on one side at a time

Therapy

Upper lobe bronchiectasis, i.e. following tuberculosis, requires no specific therapy because it drains spontaneously by gravity. The commonest clinical problem is that of middle lobe, lingula or lower lobe bronchiectasis. Therapy is as described in the following paragraphs.

Postural drainage
Postural drainage should be performed by the patient for 15–20 minutes twice daily, after initial tuition by a physiotherapist. The affected lobes are positioned uppermost to allow gravitational forces to work.

Physiotherapy
Chest percussion and vibration is performed to enable further mucus and sputum drainage.

Antibiotics
These are prescribed according to bacterial sensitivities, but whilst these are awaited, oral ampicillin 500 mg 6-hourly, or oxytetracycline 250 mg 6-hourly (not in women of child-bearing age or children because of teeth discolouration), or cotrimoxazole (960 mg 12-hourly) are all suitable. These should be started early in any infective episode. Recently, high-dose amoxycillin 3 g 12-hourly has been recommended.

Bronchodilators
β_2 adrenergic agonists, such as salbutamol, fenoterol or terbutaline, may be helpful, particularly in patients with associated asthma or aspergillosis. They are given preferably by nebulization or metered dose inhaler.

5.0 Some important diseases

5.4 Bronchiectasis

Steroids
Steroids are essential in bronchopulmonary aspergillosis to
obtain rapid clearing of the segmental infiltrates, thus leaving
the least residual damage. The initial dose is 30 mg daily until
the pulmonary shadow disappears and bronchodilation occurs,
then the dose should be gradually reduced. A maintenance
dose of 5–10 mg daily may be required to prevent recurrent
attacks and reduce the risk of residual bronchiectasis.

Bronchoscopy
Bronchoscopy may be required for extraction of mucus or
mycelial plugs, or for bronchial toilet if physiotherapy has
failed.

Surgery
Segmental resection or lobectomy can be considered if very
localized disease is seen on the bronchogram and medical
therapy has been unsuccessful. However, localized disease is
the exception rather than the rule. Recurrent severe
haemoptysis is another indication for surgery.

5.5 Tuberculosis

Types

Primary tuberculosis
The primary complex is a mid-zone (Ghon) focus with hilar
lymphadenopathy. It is usually asymptomatic but may be
detected on a routine chest X-ray, e.g. on contact tracing.
However, it may progress to:
1. bronchial spread — either obstruction of a bronchus or
   endobronchial rupture
2. pleural effusion
3. blood spread
   (a) miliary tuberculosis
   (b) meningitis
4. bone, joint or genito-urinary disease
5. post-primary tuberculosis, caused by breakdown of the
   primary lesions

1–3 normally manifest themselves within a year of infection. 4
may not occur until 10–15 years later.

5.0 Some important diseases

5.5 Tuberculosis

Post-primary tuberculosis
This is the commonest type of adult tuberculosis. The classical form of the disease (consumption, pthysis) starting with an infiltrate in the upper lobe, progressing to cavitation or healing by fibrosis or calcification. The posterior segment of the upper lobes or apical segment of the lower lobes are the areas most commonly affected.

Clinical features

The physician must be constantly aware of the possibility of tuberculosis because of its wide variety of presentations.

At-risk groups
- Asians or East Africans (who often develop the disease within a few years of arriving in the UK). In these cases the organism is usually an Asian strain.
- Alcoholics
- 'Down and outs' due to poor housing conditions, overcrowding and malnutrition
- Institution dwellers — those living in working men's hostels, prisons and mental hospitals
- Medical laboratory workers
- Doctors and nurses
- Teachers
- The elderly — possibly due to diminishing T-cell function
- Very young children, if the mother is affected, due to close maternal contact and an immature immune system

Common symptoms and signs
70% of cases are pulmonary and 30% extrapulmonary:
- Pulmonary — upper lobe infiltrate (Fig. 105) with or without cavitation. History of malaise, fever, weight loss, cough, sputum, haemoptysis
- Glandular — commonest in Asians. Palpable nodes in neck, axilla or inguinal regions
- Hilar and mediastinal node enlargement may be seen on routine chest X-ray (Fig. 106). These patients may have malaise, weight loss and fever, or be asymptomatic
- Pleural. After an initial pleurisy, there may be fever followed by shortness of breath due to the formation of a pleural effusion

194

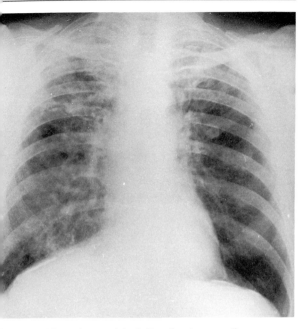

Fig. 105 *Bilateral upper lobe infiltration due to active tuberculosis.*

Rarer symptoms and signs

Tuberculous pneumonia in lobes other than the upper or apical lower — cough, sputum, fever, prostration

Meningitis — headache, fever, neck stiffness, vomiting, confusion

Bone and joint tuberculosis — vertebral (Pott's disease) or other bones and joints — local pain, neurological symptoms and signs

Erythema nodosum

Miliary tuberculosis — lungs, liver, spleen, meninges, choroid (Fig. 107), bone marrow — patient is often febrile and moribund

Phlyctenular conjunctivitis

Renal and genital tract — pyuria, fever, sterility, testicular swelling

5.5 Tuberculosis

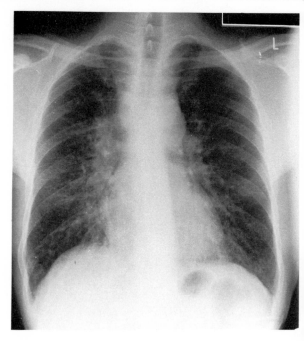

Fig. 106 *Mediastinal lymphadenopathy and miliary interstitial nodules in the lung fields due to tuberculosis.*

- Gastrointestinal — ileum and peritoneum in particular, diarrhoea, abdominal pain, ascites
- Tuberculoma — lung (coin lesion on chest X-ray) or brain, symptoms and signs of an intracerebral tumour
- Skin — Bazin's disease, lupus vulgaris (Figs 108 and 109) or erythema nodosum

Investigations

Diagnosis depends upon identifying acid-fast bacilli (*Mycobacterium tuberculosis*), either on direct smear (Ziehl-Neelsen or auramine stain) or culture (Lowenstein-Jensen medium after 2–6 weeks), of one of the following:
- sputum

5.5 Tuberculosis

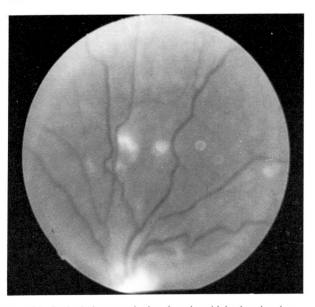

Fig. 107 *Retinal photograph showing choroidal tubercles due to miliary tuberculosis.*

- bronchial aspirates from bronchoscopic lavage
- gastric washings
- lymph node biopsy
- bone marrow aspirate
- liver biopsy
- pleural biopsy
- cerebrospinal fluid
- other histological specimens

The typical histology is that of caseating granulomata containing epithelioid giant cells. Tuberculin tests (Mantoux, Heaf and Tine) are usually positive in very dilute strengths, except in the extremely ill where they may be negative.

Therapy

Anti-tuberculous chemotherapy
Classical chemotherapy comprised streptomycin, isoniazid and

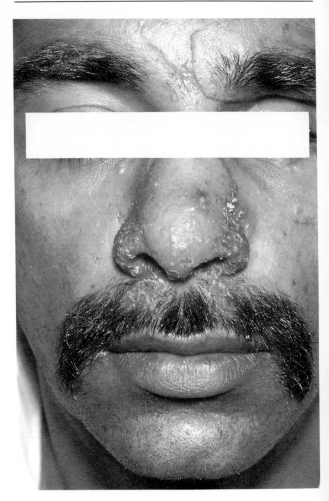

Fig. 108 *Lupus vulgaris.*

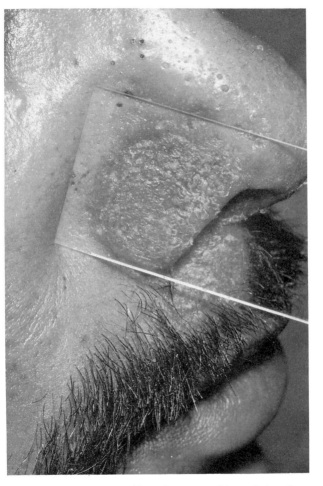

Fig. 109 *Lupus vulgaris with a microscope slide applied to the skin demonstrating an apple-jelly-like appearance.*

para-aminosalicylic acid (PAS) for 18 months. Because streptomycin needs to be injected and may cause otovestibular toxicity in patients and skin sensitivity in the nursing staff handling it, and PAS (only a weak drug) frequently causes indigestion, these drugs are now used less in the UK. However, as they are cheap, some underdeveloped countries still use them.

Current antituberculous therapy
This consists of rifampicin 450 mg (wt. < 50 kg) or 600 mg (wt. > 50 kg) together with isoniazid 300 mg and ethambutol 15 mg/kg. These are all given once daily in the morning on an empty stomach. In addition, pyridoxine 10 mg daily is given to malnourished patients to prevent isoniazid peripheral neuropathy. Before commencement of therapy the following must be done:

- baseline liver function tests in case of later rifampicin or isoniazid hepatitis
- check visual fields, acuity and colour vision, in case of visual disturbances with ethambutol (occurring in 2%). Warn patient to stop ethambutol if any visual disturbance occurs
- warn the patient that his urine and stools will become orange/red with rifampicin treatment
- notify the patient to the District Community Physician or equivalent using the appropriate form

All 3 drugs are given for the first 2 months or until the drug sensitivities of the organism are known if this is earlier when ethambutol is stopped (if the organism is sensitive to rifampicin and isoniazid). The other 2 drugs are continued for a further 7 months. Patients with bone TB are usually treated for a total of 18 months.

Two antituberculous drugs are given to avoid the emergence of drug-resistant mycobacteria (currently 3% — mainly isoniazid resistant). Combination preparations containing rifampicin and isoniazid, or isoniazid and ethambutol are available, so that the number of tablets taken can be reduced.

Antituberculous therapy — the future
There is growing evidence that antituberculous therapy can be shortened to 6 months by the addition of a fourth drug — pyrazinamide (1.5 g/d wt < 50 kg; 2.0 g/d wt 50–74 kg or 2.5 g/d wt > 74 kg) — for the first 2 months of treatment.

5.5 Tuberculosis

Table 10 Side-effects of antituberculous drugs.

	Rifampicin	Isoniazid	Ethambutol	Pyrazinamide	Streptomycin	Capreomycin	Cycloserine
Nausea	+	+	–	+	–	–	–
Vomiting	+	+	–	+	–	–	–
Anorexia	+	+	–	+	–	–	+
Rashes	+	+	–	+	+	+	–
Hepatitis	+	+	–	+	–	+	–
Peripheral neuropathy	–	+	–	–	–	–	–
Otovestibular toxicity	–	–	–	–	+	+	+
Arthralgia	–	–	–	+	–	–	–
Convulsions	–	+	–	–	–	–	–
Psychosis	–	+	–	–	–	–	–
Effect on the blood	Thrombocytopenic purpura	Agranulocytosis	–	Sideroblastic anaemia	–	–	–
Other effects	Oral contraceptive effectiveness reduced		Retrobulbar neuritis		Renal toxicity		

5.0 Some important diseases

5.5 Tuberculosis

Pregnancy

The best advice before prescribing antituberculous chemotherapy for a pregnant woman is to check with the information pharmacist or drug manufacturer first, because adverse reports and new knowledge are constantly being acquired. It is rare that treatment needs to be started before a careful check is made.

- Streptomycin crosses the placenta so it should not be used
- There is some evidence of teratogenicity in animals with rifampicin. In women, however, the risks of fetal abnormality or miscarriage are greater with tuberculosis than with rifampicin therapy. Therefore, although the drug should not be given if there is an alternative available, in severe life-threatening disease the drug may be used
- Isoniazid, ethambutol and PAS are safe
- Pyrazinamide is probably safe but there is little information to date

Steroids

Steroids are used in combination with antituberculous therapy to prevent residual fibrosis, initially at a dose of 20 mg/day (30–40 mg in the severely ill) in the following situations:

- meningitis
- pericarditis
- peritonitis
- pleural effusion

In severely malnourished patients, steroids may also be used as an appetite stimulant in order to achieve weight gain. They are also given to the desperately sick patient to reduce the toxicity of the disease. Once the disease is controlled (usually within 4–6 weeks) the dosage of steroids can be reduced over a month and stopped.

Follow-up

When tuberculosis is suspected it is often best to admit the patient to a hospital side ward for a few days to make the diagnosis, educate the patient about the disease and start therapy. It is important to ascertain whether the patient will be able to tolerate therapy. After discharge from hospital, patients should be seen and X-rayed at monthly intervals for the first 3 months, then at 3-monthly intervals until the end of therapy.

Patients can be discharged from follow-up 3 months after completion of chemotherapy if there are no complications. However, patients with bone or renal tuberculosis should be monitored for a longer period. This applies also to old patients who have never had adequate chemotherapy for previous TB.

In the UK, the family and contacts of patients will be traced and investigated by the local chest clinic staff through the notification system. Contacts should have chest X-rays, and Heaf or other tuberculin tests. Those patients with evidence of disease should be treated fully. In some regions those with positive Heaf tests, but with no evidence of BCG immunization or obvious current or previous infection, are given antituberculous chemoprophylaxis for 6 months (rifampicin and isoniazid). Antituberculous chemoprophylaxis is also given to known tuberculin converters (except if this has been caused by BCG vaccination).

Prevention

Vaccination against tuberculosis is by injection of the Bacillus Calmette-Guérin (BCG) in order to raise T-cell-mediated immunity. This bacillus is a strain of bovine *Mycobacterium tuberculosis* which has lost its virulence.

In the UK, BCG vaccination reduces the risk of tuberculosis in the population by 80% over 10 years. It is given at birth to children of mothers who have tuberculosis and in areas with a high incidence of tuberculosis. Otherwise it is given to children aged 12–13 years.

5.6 Chronic bronchitis

Chronic bronchitis is recognized by the presence of a cough productive of sputum on most days of 3 successive months in 2 consecutive years. It should be differentiated from emphysema which is a pathological diagnosis involving dilation of the terminal airspaces and destruction of alveolar walls. Both conditions may coexist to a greater or lesser extent in the same patient, producing a spectrum of chronic obstructive airways disease (COAD), known as chronic obstructive pulmonary disease (COPD) in the USA.

Causes

- Tobacco smoking
- Atmospheric pollution

Clinical features

Symptoms
- Cough — beginning as a 'smoker's cough'
- Sputum — mucoid but purulent in infective exacerbations
- Wheeze — the patient is aware of noisy breathing
- Shortness of breath — gradual reduction in exercise tolerance

Signs
There may be none early in the disease. Gradually one or more of the following occur:
- obvious dyspnoea
- use of accessory muscles of respiration
- diminished but symmetrical chest movement
- percussion note — resonant or hyper-resonant
- diminished breath sounds — all zones
- wheezes (rhonchi) — usually expiratory but may also be inspiratory. In very severe disease the chest may be quiet, there being inadequate airflow to cause turbulence necessary to produce wheezes
- cyanosis may be present late in the disease
- finger clubbing does *not* occur

Complications

Acute exacerbations
With or without evidence of bacterial infection

Cor pulmonale
Progressive pulmonary hypertension due to hypoxia and hypercapnia leads to right ventricular enlargement and failure with raised jugular venous pressure, hepatomegaly and peripheral oedema.

5.0 Some important diseases

5.6 Chronic bronchitis

Respiratory failure
Hypoxia and CO_2 retention — type II respiratory failure
'The blue bloater'

Polycythaemia
Chronic hypoxia causes increased renal erythropoietin secretion
and hence bone marrow stimulation.

Lung cancer
There is double the incidence of lung cancer in male bronchitics
(common cause — smoking).

Pneumothorax
Ruptured bulla can occur if there is coexistent emphysema.

Investigations

Full blood count
If O_2 saturation is chronically less than 92%, secondary
polycythaemia may occur.

Chest X-ray
There are no specific changes of chronic bronchitis, although
there may be hyperinflation. An X-ray is essential to exclude a
coexistent carcinoma.

ECG
Right atrial and ventricular hypertrophy and strain occur as cor
pulmonale develops.

Sputum
During infective episodes, common bacterial pathogens are
H. influenzae and *Strep. pneumoniae*.

Lung function tests
There is an obstructive ventilatory defect with very little
reversibility to β agonists (up to 20%). The airways resistance
is high leading to a high residual volume. The gas transfer is
relatively well preserved unless there is coexisting emphysema.

Blood gases
Hypoxia occurs early in the disease. Later there is both hypoxia
and hypercapnia. Ventilatory response to rising CO_2 is
abnormally blunted, but the hypoxic response is normal.

5.0 Some important diseases

5.6 Chronic bronchitis

Therapy — routine out-patient

Smoking
The 2 main causative factors are cigarette smoking and generalized or local atmospheric pollution. Cigarette smoking should be actively discouraged in order to stop the deterioration in lung function. If smoking continues, deterioration will inevitably continue.

Bronchodilators
Although by definition airways obstruction can only be reversed by 20% at most, this small amount can be valuable and make all the difference to the more severely affected patient. Inhaled β_2 agonists — salbutamol 200 μg or terbutaline 500 μg or fenoterol 400 μg 6-hourly — are useful. Anticholinergics such as ipratropium bromide 40 μg 6-hourly may also be tried.

Steroids
Oral and inhaled steroids play no part in the routine maintenance therapy of chronic bronchitis. However, whenever there is doubt as to whether a patient might be a chronic asthmatic rather than a chronic bronchitic with irreversible airways obstruction, a 2-week trial of oral prednisone 30 mg daily should be tried to assess the maximum reversibility and hence exclude asthma.

Mucolytics
There are numerous mucolytic agents, none of which has convincing beneficial actions.

Opiates and sedatives
These are to be avoided because they depress respiratory drive.

Antibiotics
In acute infective exacerbations a broad-spectrum oral antibiotic such as ampicillin (250–500 mg 6-hourly), or oxytetracycline (250–500 mg 6-hourly), or cotrimoxazole 960 mg 12-hourly should be given to cover *H. influenzae* and the *Strep.* pneumoniae whilst sputum culture results are awaited. Long-term antibiotics are not needed as they may lead to superinfection with antibiotic-resistant organisms. However,

patients should have a supply at home to take immediately their sputum becomes purulent.

Diuretics
Cor pulmonale can be controlled by frusemide alone or in combination with amiloride, the dose being regulated according to requirements.

Digoxin
This is required only to control atrial fibrillation.

Oxygen
There is now evidence that life may be prolonged by continuous low-dose oxygen (24–28%) for 15 hours each night. This delays the onset of pulmonary hypertension.

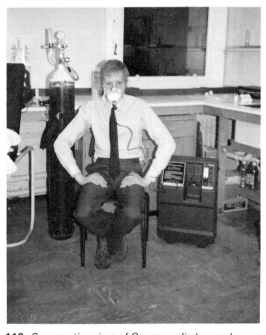

Fig. 110 *Comparative sizes of Oxygen cylinders and concentrators.*

Oxygen can be provided by cylinders or, more economically and safely, by domiciliary oxygen concentrators (Fig. 110).

Therapy — severe acute exacerbations

Hospitalization

Controlled oxygen therapy
Controlled oxygen therapy is 24% initially, increasing according to blood gas results (check Pa_{CO_2} does not rise, i.e. worsening alveolar hypoventilation). Care is taken to avoid depressing respiration by totally abolishing the hypoxic drive because the patient may be insensitive to rises in Pa_{CO_2}.

Broad-spectrum antibiotics
Broad-spectrum antibiotics are administered as ampicillin 500 mg 6-hourly, or oxytetracycline 500 mg 6-hourly, or cotrimoxazole 960 mg 12-hourly.

Physiotherapy
Physiotherapy is instituted to aid expectoration of sputum.

Bronchodilators
Bronchodilation is by i.v. infusion of aminophylline 0.5 mg/kg/h in 5% dextrose regulated by blood theophylline levels. In addition to nebulized salbutamol 5 mg or terbutaline 5 mg or fenoterol 2.5 mg 6-hourly.

Diuretics
Diuretics are given for cor pulmonale — frusemide alone or with amiloride.

Digoxin
Digoxin is used to control atrial fibrillation (if present).

Respiratory failure
Doxapram infusion and artificial ventilation may be indicated see **6.2**.

5.7 Emphysema

Causes

Emphysema is primarily a pathological diagnosis which is suggested rather than proven during life. There are four pathological types, but all have the same clinical features:

- panlobular (panacinar)
- proximal acinar (centriacinar, centrilobular)
- paraseptal (periacinar or distal acinar)
- irregular

Often two or more types are found in the same patient. Chronic bronchitis is very commonly associated with emphysema. Smoking causes proximal acinar emphysema. Alpha$_1$ antitrypsin deficiency panlobular disease. Panlobular disease is also associated with obliterative bronchiolitis, e.g. MacLeod's syndrome (unilateral emphysema following childhood bronchiolitis).

Clinical features

Symptoms
- Shortness of breath — at first on exercise, then later even at rest, this may be very distressing to the patient
- Cough and sputum are associated with coexistent chronic bronchitis, but may be absent in 'pure' emphysema
- weight loss

Signs
'The pink puffer' appearance is classical with symptoms as follows:
- thinness
- obvious dyspnoea
- pursed lip expiration
- using accessory muscles of respiration
- hyperinflated chest
- hyper-resonant percussion note
- diminished breath sounds in all areas
- the chest is often quiet but expiratory wheezes can be heard, particularly on forced expiration
- finger clubbing does *not* occur

5.0 Some important diseases

5.7 Emphysema

Complications

Acute infective episodes
Acute infective episodes will occur particularly if there is associated chronic bronchitis.

Cor pulmonale and respiratory failure
These are often precipitated by infection.

Pneumothorax
A small pneumothorax caused by rupture of an emphysematous bulla may be life-threatening in severe emphysema.

Lung cancer
Lung cancer may be a complication of emphysema because of their shared aetiology — smoking.

Investigations

Chest X-ray
Hyperinflation, low flat diaphragms, narrow mediastinum, small 'tear-drop' heart. Absence of lung marker vessels in the peripheral third of the lung fields. Bullae may be obvious. Check for pneumothorax or coexistent cancer.

CT scan of chest
This is rarely necessary but will show bullae and greater destruction than suspected on the plain chest X-ray.

Lung function tests
Irreversible obstructive defect may be present with hyperinflation and gas trapping. There will be very low gas transfer. There is extremely little, if any, response to bronchodilators. Flow volume loop shows 'early airways collapse' with relative preservation of peak flow.

Blood gases
Pa_{O_2} is relatively well preserved. Pa_{CO_2} is low due to hyperventilation. There is a normal ventilatory response to CO_2 and hypoxia.

Sputum
Common pathogens in infective episodes include *H. influenzae* and the Pneumococcus.

Serum alpha₁ antitrypsin

This should be measured in patients under 50 with basal emphysema and in any non-smoker with emphysema.

Therapy

There is no very effective therapy, however, the following alternatives may be tried.

Stopping smoking

If the patient stops smoking, this will decrease the rate of decline of lung function and stabilize the situation. If he continues to smoke, the outlook is poor.

Bronchodilator therapy

As in chronic bronchitis, a very small amount of improvement may be possible with either β agonist or anticholinergics

Antibiotics

Antibiotics may be used for acute infective episodes.

Oxygen

In acute exacerbations, 35% or higher concentration may be given from the onset as the response to CO_2 is normal, hence it does not matter removing the hypoxic drive. Blood gases should be measured as a precaution to check that the $Paco_2$ is not rising. Domiciliary oxygen may be of considerable help, at least symptomatically.

Steroids

Steroids play no part in the management of emphysema once asthma has been excluded by a 14-day course of oral prednisone 30 mg daily.

Promethazine

Promethazine may reduce the subjective feeling of breathlessness but does not improve lung function.

Diuretics

For preterminal cor pulmonale diuretics may be given.

Opiates and other sedatives
These are to be avoided.

5.8 Alpha$_1$ antitrypsin deficiency

Alpha$_1$ antitrypsin is a potent inhibitor of the trypsin-like enzymes, for example, elastase, which are released from pulmonary inflammatory cells in response to infection or insults such as inhalation of cigarette smoke. Alpha$_1$ antitrypsin deficiency leads to panlobular emphysema.

The severest form of the disease occurs in the homozygote (PiZZ) patients who have alpha$_1$ antitrypsin levels 15–30% of normal (PiMM). Heterozygotes (PiMZ) have levels 50–80% of normal. Only the smokers in this group (PiMZ) have problems. The incidence of the Z allele in the population is 3–5%. PiZZ occurs in 1:5000 of the population.

Clinical features

- Progressive shortness of breath
- Young patients (60% of the emphysematous patients under 40 years of age)
- Severe emphysema (Fig. 111) — mainly basal
- May be non-smokers

Complications

- Pneumothorax — if an emphysematous bulla ruptures
- Respiratory failure
- Hepatic cirrhosis both in children and adults

Therapy

Patients with alpha$_1$ antitrypsin must be advised to:
- stop smoking
- avoid polluted atmospheres and dusty jobs
- have their relatives checked for alpha$_1$ antitrypsin deficiency so that they can also be advised appropriately

5.9 Asthma

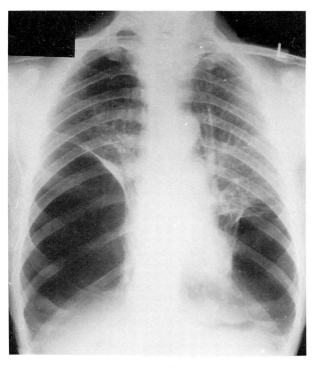

Fig. 111 *Large bilateral basal bullae due to emphysema caused by alpha $_1$ antitrypsin deficiency.*

5.9 Asthma

Asthma is very common, affecting up to 5% of the population. It may occur for the first time at any age, but the peak incidence is in young children.

Clinical features

Asthma is characterized by reversible airways obstruction. There is no time limit to this reversibility, it can be within a few minutes or take a few weeks or more. The amount of improvement in FEV_1, or PEFR necessary for the reversibility to be significant is arbitrarily taken as 20%. Lesser amounts of reversibility can be observed in non-asthmatic chronic bronchitics.

The following factors contribute to the airways obstruction in asthma:
- bronchial smooth muscle spasm
- bronchial wall oedema
- increased mucus production

Common symptoms
Symptoms may occur spontaneously or they may be related to the seasons of the year, or to specific allergen exposure or exercise. Typical symptoms are:
- episodic shortness of breath
- audible wheezing
- cough
- sputum production

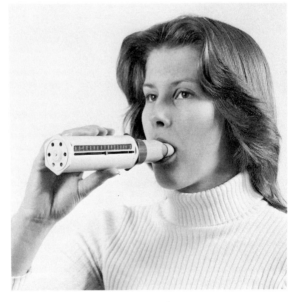

Fig. 112 *Peak flow gauge in operation.*

5.9 Asthma

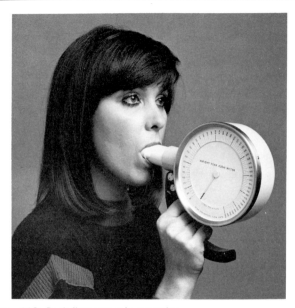

Fig. 113 *Peak flow meter in operation.*

Common signs of severe asthma
- Visible dyspnoea and tachypnoea with the use of accessory muscles of respiration
- Tachycardia
- Pulsus paradoxus ($> 10-15$ mmHg)
- Hyperinflated chest
- Hyper-resonant chest
- Diminished air entry — symmetrical
- Expiratory ± inspiratory wheezes (rhonchi)

Very serious signs
- Cyanosis
- Silent chest — inadequate air flow in or out of chest to generate wheezes
- Hypotension

Assessing the severity of an attack
The following variables are used to assess the severity of the asthmatic attack both initially and at regular intervals to monitor the response to treatment.

5.0 Some important diseases

5.9 Asthma

- FEV_1 or peak flow rate
- pulse rate
- pulsus paradoxus
- blood gases

It should be noted that all of these are objective measurements. Subjective variables such as the patient's feeling of dyspnoea and the wheeziness of his chest play little part in managing the acute attack.

Investigations

Respiratory function tests
Respiratory function tests are necessary both to confirm the diagnosis of asthma and to monitor response to therapy. The tests show reversible airways obstruction ($\downarrow FEV_1/FVC$ %) with large lungs ($\uparrow TLC$; total lung capacity) and gas trapping ($\uparrow RV$; residual volume) when there is an asthma attack; gas transfer is normal or raised.

Asthma is an episodic disease, and between attacks the patient's lung function can be completely normal. The change in peak flow rate or FEV_1 after 5 minutes of vigorous exercise and during the recovery phase (30 minutes) is a very valuable test in bringing to light those patients with exercise-induced asthma; deterioration of over 20% is diagnostic. This test can be repeated on subsequent days after pretreatment with sodium cromoglycate or salbutamol to see whether the therapy is effective. Another useful test is to ask the patient to record his PEFR at home twice daily for 2 or 3 weeks; again any variability of over 20% is diagnostic.

Allergy tests
All asthmatics should have skin prick tests performed to detect allergies to the common allergens, e.g. house dust mite (*D. pteronyssinus*), cat fur, feathers, grasses, dog fur, eggs, milk, moulds, trees, house dust, aspergillus, flowers. These tests should be read after 10–20 minutes. If positive responses are obtained to the mixes, individual tests can be performed for each of the 4 or 5 constituents. The aspergillus test should be examined again 4–6 hours later for a delayed type III response. The weal rather than the erythema is taken as the response. Sometimes responses of 1 cm or more are obtained.

Radioallergosorbent tests (RAST)
RAST tests detect specific serum IgE antibodies against common inhaled allergens. These correlate well with the skin tests. However, they take longer, are more expensive and add little further information to that obtained from the skin tests. RAST tests to foods are also available. As yet, the significance of a positive food RAST is unknown.

Aspergillus precipitins
These are often found in bronchopulmonary aspergillosis.

Chest X-ray
Usually, the X-ray will be normal apart from showing large lungs with low diaphragms, but it is essential in an acute asthma attack to exclude a pneumothorax, mediastinal emphysema or pneumonia.

Sputum
The presence of eosinophils is often commented upon, in both allergic (atopic) and non allergic (intrinsic) asthma. A Gram stain and culture is performed to search for bacterial infection as the precipitating cause of an attack (20% or fewer). Aspergillus hyphae may be identified in exacerbations of aspergillosis.

Blood gases
Arterial blood gas tensions are very useful in assessing the severity of an attack (Fig. 114), and the response to therapy. However, lung function tests are easier to perform and are more acceptable to the patient. The Pao_2 falls progressively with increasing severity of an attack, because of ventilation perfusion (V/Q) mismatch. The $Paco_2$ initially falls because the patient hyperventilates: as the severity of the attack increases the airways narrow further, so ventilation is gradually impaired, causing the $Paco_2$ to rise first back into the normal range and then later to become elevated. This is an extremely serious situation, and may well necessitate artificial ventilation. Associated with the usual low $Paco_2$ there is a respiratory alkalosis. Blood gases often take 10–14 days longer than the FEV_1 or PEFR to return to normal after resolution of an asthma attack (due to the mucus plugging causing V/Q mismatch).

5.9 Asthma

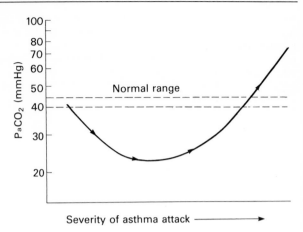

Fig. 114 *Changes in the arterial Paco$_2$ with increasing severity of an asthma attack. Initially there is a low Paco$_2$ due to hyperventilation as the airways obstruction worsens so there is alveolar hypoventilation and a rise in the Paco$_2$. A normal or raised Paco$_2$ in an asthma attack is a serious sign.*

Blood count
Eosinophilia is often noted in atopic asthma.

Electrolytes
Serum potassium should be checked (it is often reduced with a respiratory alkalosis) to minimize the risk of cardiac arrhythmias with bronchodilators. (β agonists also cause hypokalaemia.)

Immunoglobulins
Elevated serum IgE levels are found in allergic individuals.

Prevention

Antigen avoidance
Skin tests identify *possible* not *definite* causes of asthma. Once allergens have been identified, specific advice can be given about avoidance for at least a trial period. This may be relatively easy, e.g. avoiding certain animals; or more difficult, e.g. avoiding house dust mites (Fig. 115). The advice given to patients allergic to the latter is to vacuum their homes as much

5.9 Asthma

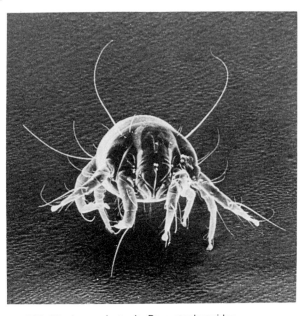

Fig. 115 *The house dust mite* Dermatophagoides pteronyssinus.

as possible, including mattresses and bedding, and to use synthetic bedding and pillows. Wrapping the mattress in a plastic sheet is the only effective way of reducing antigen exposure from it. It only takes about 6 months for the house dust mite to get up to 'full strength' in a new mattress.

Drug avoidance
Patients who are allergic to aspirin should also avoid other analgesics, such as indomethacin and paracetamol, which can also precipitate asthma. Asthmatics should avoid contraindicated drugs, particularly sedatives which depress respiration, and non-selective β-adrenergic blocking drugs such as propranolol which cause bronchospasm. Even 'selective' β-blockers (e.g. atenolol, metoprolol) should be used only with great caution.

5.9 Asthma

Desensitization

Numerous preparations are available which claim to desensitize atopic individuals. Repeated injections are given to try and raise blocking IgG antibody, with limited success. However, there are 2 occasions when desensitization might be worth trying. One is when teenage children with pollen hay fever are taking exams in the summer and their performance in these is likely to be affected, either by asthma or hay fever or by the side-effects of the antihistamines taken for their symptoms. In this group, desensitization should be commenced 2 years before major exams and continued for 5 years. Injections begin in February and finish in April each year.

Another group where desensitization may be worth trying are the adult atopic asthmatics in whom all other therapy has failed. A 5-year course should also be given, again from February to April each year.

Care should be taken with desensitization, as fatalities have been recorded due to anaphylaxis. The patient should be observed for 30 minutes after each injection. Adrenaline and hydrocortisone injections should be immediately available should resuscitation be required.

Therapy

It should be remembered that approximately 1500 asthmatics die from the disease each year — these are often young people. With good, adequate treatment and by allowing patients to refer themselves directly to the hospital, many of these deaths might be avoided. Discharge of asthmatics from casualty departments after a single bolus of i.v. aminophylline should be discouraged as most of these patients require admission for proper control of their asthma. A good indication of when a patient's asthma is out of control is when he is getting 'morning dips' of peak flow rate sufficient to wake him in the early hours or to make him very breathless on waking. If these dips are occurring, vigorous therapy is required.

Large 'dips' also occur as the patient is recovering from an acute asthma attack and the patient should not be discharged until these large oscillations have disappeared.

5.9 Asthma

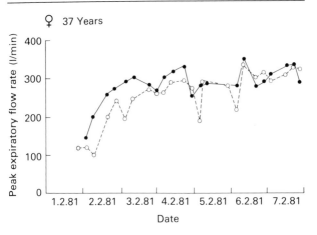

Fig. 116 *Peak flow chart showing recovery from an acute asthma attack; o —— o, before and •——•, after, salbutamol inhalation.*

Mild asthma

Some patients have very occasional problems for which the symptomatic use of metered dose inhalers of either salbutamol, terbutaline, or fenoterol may be recommended. Another group of patients has symptoms limited to one season of the year (e.g. pollen season). For these patients sodium cromoglycate 20 mg 6-hourly is given for the month before symptoms are expected to occur and continued regularly until the pollen season is over. A β_2 adrenergic inhaler is also given in case some symptoms still occur.

Moderate asthma

For allergic patients, sodium cromoglycate 20 mg 6-hourly to avert attacks is the treatment of choice, supplemented by a salbutamol inhaler for symptomatic relief 200 µg 6-hourly. If these prove inadequate, substitute an inhaled steroid, e.g. beclomethasone 2 puffs (100 µg) 6-hourly in place of sodium cromoglycate. Few non-allergic patients respond to sodium cromoglycate, thus maintenance is with an inhaled steroid and β-agonist.

5.0 Some important diseases

5.9 Asthma

Severe asthma

For patients who are inadequately controlled using inhaled β_2 stimulants and either sodium cromoglycate or low-dose inhaled steroids, try one or more of the following:

- high-dose steroid inhalers — becloforte or budesonide
- ipratropium inhaler 40 μg 6-hourly
- oral theophyllines — slow-release 12-hourly — control dose according to blood levels
- oral steroids

Any asthmatic who is to be given oral steroids needs the following:

- questioning about peptic ulceration — give enteric-coated tablets if there is a history of indigestion. Do not start steroids in a patient with active ulceration.
- urine checking regularly to exclude diabetes
- blood pressure check
- steroid card
- chest X-ray to exclude active tuberculosis

Systemic steroids should be reserved for the following situations.

(a) Severe persistent attacks. A short course of oral prednisone is given, 30 mg daily until the attack is over (usually 3–7 days), and continued at this dose for a further 3 days, then reduced by 5 mg per day every 3 days until the steroids are stopped. If symptoms begin to recur, the dose should not be lowered so rapidly. Inhaled steroids are continued on a regular dose throughout.

(b) Diagnostic trial of steroids. In patients with chronic airflow obstruction, assess baseline function (PEFR or FEV_1) over several days and then give oral prednisone 30 mg daily, and follow changes in lung function. An improvement in the FEV_1 or PEFR of greater than 20% is diagnostic of asthma. It is rarely worth giving more than 14 days' trial. Other bronchodilators are given simultaneously to assess the maximum possible reversibility. Once maximum improvement has been obtained, oral steroids should be rapidly discontinued over 1–2 weeks and inhaled steroids substituted if the patient has been shown to be asthmatic. If not, neither oral nor inhaled steroids are indicated.

(c) Continuation therapy. A few patients cannot be managed on inhaled steroids even when given in high doses and require an oral dose. This is rarely more than 5.0–7.5 mg prednisone daily.

Special points on out-patient therapy

Check inhaler technique. This is poor in many patients. All patients must be shown how to use inhalers properly (placebo inhalers are readily available from all manufacturers). For patients who are unable to use metered-dose inhalers, even after tuition, prescribe a dry powder device (salbutamol or fenoterol) or a spacer (terbutaline).

Check patient is using drugs regularly. Poor patient compliance often occurs either because the patient does not understand why he needs drugs such as inhaled steroids or sodium cromoglycate which give no immediate bronchodilation, or because he is being asked to take too many drugs. The maximum a patient can reasonably be expected to take regularly is 2 inhalers and 1 type of tablet; therefore, try to simplify treatment whenever possible.

Always ask about exercise-induced asthma. This can be very limiting, especially in the young. It often responds to β_2 agonist or sodium cromoglycate inhaled 5–10 minutes before exercise.

Other asthma treatments
- Breathing exercises
- Hypnosis
- Antihistamines
- Inhalation of negative ions

There is no definite objective evidence that any of these are helpful in asthma.

Treatment of angina and hypertension in asthmatics
'Selective' β-blockers such as metoprolol and atenolol are *less* likely to induce bronchospasm than the more selective agents such as propranolol but even these drugs must be given with *extreme caution*. In patients with coexistent airways obstruction treat angina with nitrites in the first place, if these are inadequate use a calcium antagonist:
- nifedipine 10 mg 8-hourly, or

5.9 Asthma

- lidoflazine 120 mg daily initially, rising over 3 weeks to 120 mg 8-hourly, or
- verapamil 80 mg 8-hourly

Hypertension in asthma should be treated initially by diet, weight loss and a thiazide diuretic such as bendrofluazide 5 mg daily. If this is inadequate add either methyldopa (250 mg 12-hourly initially) or nifedipine 10 mg 8-hourly or hydralazine (25 mg 12-hourly initially)

Emergency asthma therapy

Immediate therapy
1. Assess severity of attack — obtain baseline readings for the 4 'p's:
   - *p*ulse rate > 120 beats/min
   - *p*eak flow rate < 120 l/min
   - Po_2 ↓ + Pco_2 — normal or elevated
   - *p*ulsus paradoxus > 20 mmHg

   } any are criteria for hospitalization.
2. Give 35% oxygen continuously.
3. Nebulized salbutamol 5 mg over 5–10 minutes (or fenoterol (2.5 mg) or terbutaline (5 mg)).
4. i.v. aminophylline 5 mg/kg over 10 minutes (unless patient is already on theophylline preparations).
5. i.v. hydrocortisone 200 mg statim.

Continuation therapy
Repeat 4 'p's to assess the response at 20 minutes (blood gases need only be repeated if there is doubt about improvement using the other three).
1. Aminophylline 0.5 mg/kg/hr in 5% dextrose — monitored by serum theophylline levels.
2. Hydrocortisone 200 mg 6-hourly i.v. initially.
3. Oral prednisone 40 mg daily.
4. Nebulized salbutamol 5 mg 6-hourly.
5. 35% oxygen continuously.
6. Antibiotics (e.g. ampicillin 500 mg 6-hourly or cotrimoxazole 960 mg 12-hourly) only if there is evidence of bacterial infection.
7. Monitor fluid balance.

Indications for assisted ventilation
- Exhaustion and respiratory distress

5.0 Some important diseases

5.9 Asthma

- $Pao_2 < 50$ mmHg (6.5 kPa) and falling
- $Paco_2 > 50$ mmHg (6.5 kPa) and rising
- Hypotension (BP systolic < 90 mmHg)
- Respiratory (± cardiac) arrest

5.10 Carcinoma of the bronchus

Causes

Lung cancer is the commonest of all cancers in males. Although in males the incidence has levelled off, in women it is still rising. The largest aetiological factor is almost certainly cigarette smoking. The prognosis of lung cancer can only be described as appalling (only 5% overall 5 years survival). This is mainly because the presentation of the disease is often through either local or distant metastases. Little, if any, improvement has been made in the survival figures either with

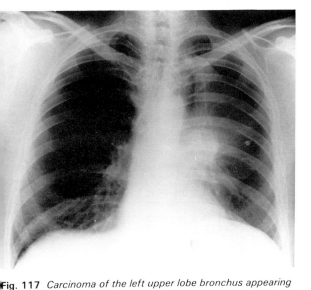

Fig. 117 *Carcinoma of the left upper lobe bronchus appearing as a left hilar mass and causing left upper lobe collapse. Note the overexpanded left lower lobe and herniation of the right upper lobe across the midline.*

225

regular (6-monthly) chest X-rays or with the introduction of the fibreoptic bronchoscope. Although the life-expectancy of patients with small cell (oat cell) tumours is improving (c. 18 months) with the development of chemotherapy, the overwhelming message to the population must be *'do not smoke'*.

Clinical features

There are a large number of symptoms with which a patient with bronchial carcinoma may present. However, occasionally tumours are detected in asymptomatic people on routine chest X-ray (mass miniature or pre-employment). The commonest clinical features are listed in the following paragraphs.

Non-specific symptoms
• Weight loss
• Poor appetite
• Malaise
• Fever

Features due to localized tumour
• Persistent cough
• Haemoptysis
• Slowly resolving pneumonia
• Lobar collapse
• Stridor (central tumours)

Features due to pleural and chest wall spread
• Pleurisy
• Pleural effusion — shortness of breath
• Pancoast tumour — Horner's syndrome together with brachial plexus invasion, pain down arm with wasting of muscles in hypothenar eminence

Features due to mediastinal spread
• Dull retrosternal ache
• Superior vena caval obstruction (Fig. 118) — swollen head and arms, prominent non-pulsatile veins in upper half of body
• Phrenic nerve palsy (Fig. 119) — sudden shortness of breath
• Recurrent laryngeal nerve palsy — hoarse voice, bovine cough

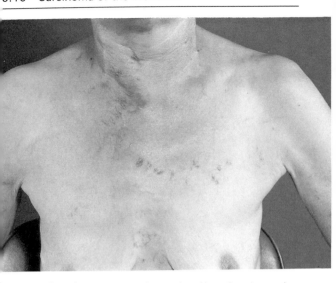

Fig. 118 *Superior vena cava obstruction. Note the engorged neck veins and the prominent superficial veins over the chest.*

- Pericardial effusion — pain ± atrial fibrillation, shortness of breath if constriction is occurring, pulsus paradoxus

Features due to distant metastases

Cerebral features are:
- headaches, neck stiffness and vomiting — caused by raised intracranial pressure
- Jacksonian (focal) fits
- focal weakness or sensory loss
- transient ischaemic attacks
- behavioural changes (frontal lobe secondaries)

Hepatic features are:
- hepatomegaly (abdominal swelling)
- jaundice (rare)

Lymph nodes. These may feature:
- enlarged glands particularly in the neck, axtillae and supraclavicular fossae

227

5.10 Carcinoma of the bronchus

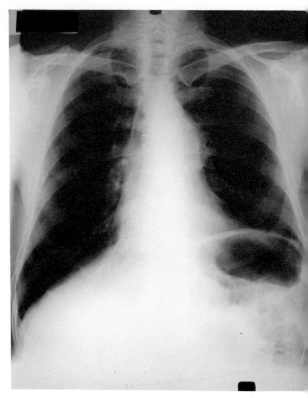

Fig. 119 *Elevated left hemidiaphragm due to a phrenic nerve palsy caused by spread from a left upper lobe carcinoma.*

Bones may display the following features:
- local pain
- pathological fractures — through a metastasis

Adrenals. These may be affected and cause:
- Addison's disease

Skin may feature:
- painless nodule (metastasis)

5.0 Some important diseases

5.10 Carcinoma of the bronchus

Features due to non-metastatic manifestations

Skeletal features are:
- clubbing of the fingers and toes
- wrist and ankle pain — hypertrophic pulmonary osteoarthropathy

Endocrine features are:
- inappropriate ADH secretion — confusion and fits
- hypercalcaemia — due to ectopic PTH secretion, usually squamous cell carcinoma.

Cases of ectopic secretion of almost every hormone by oat cell cancers have been described. The commonest are:
- Cushing's syndrome — ectopic ACTH secretion
- thyrotoxicosis — ectopic TSH secretion

Neuromuscular defects due to non-metastatic manifestations are:
- dementia
- cerebellar degeneration causing incoordination
- peripheral neuropathies — numbness and weakness in the limbs starting peripherally and spreading centrally
- myopathy
- myasthenia
- polymyositis

Common signs
From the list of possible presentations due to local or metastatic disease the clinical signs may be extremely varied. However, common physical signs include the following:
- weight loss
- clubbing of the fingers and toes
- lymphadenopathy — neck, supraclavicular fossae or axillae — due to metastases
- chest signs — often there are none. There may be a very large tumour seen on X-ray, yet no detectable clinical signs, but there may be signs either of a pneumonia or collapse distal to obstruction of a lobar bronchus by tumour or signs of a pleural effusion if the pleura is invaded
- cardiovascular — atrial fibrillation or pericardial rub — with pericardial involvement
- abdomen — hepatomegaly due to metastases

5.10 Carcinoma of the bronchus

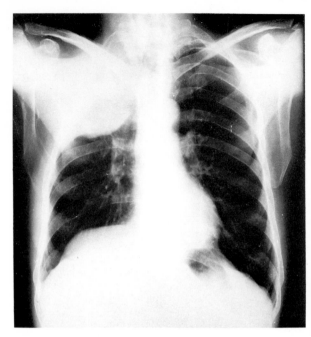

Fig. 120 *Carcinoma of the right upper lobe showing local invasion and destruction of the ribs.*

Investigations

These are directed firstly towards obtaining a histological diagnosis of the primary tumour, and secondly, towards defining the extent of local and metastatic spread to assess operability.

Routine
The following routine examinations or tests should be made:
- chest X-ray, PA and lateral — this may show a hilar mass, a cavitating lesion, a peripheral solitary coin lesion or lobar collapse/consolidation
- full blood count and ESR — raised white cell count with bacterial superinfection, non-specific elevation of ESR, leukoerythroblastic anaemia with bone marrow infiltration

5.10 Carcinoma of the bronchus

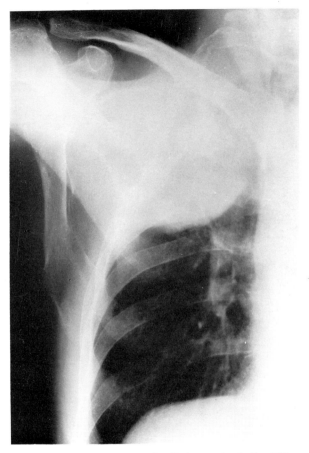

Fig. 121 *Tomogram showing the rib destruction in Fig. 120.*

- urea and electrolytes — hyponatraemia with inappropriate ADH secretion
- liver function tests — elevated alkaline phosphatase with liver (or bone) metastases
- sputum for cytology on 3 occasions may be diagnostic
- sputum for culture including acid fast bacilli (AFB) — to pick

231

up bacterial superinfection and aid in the differential
diagnosis
- lung function tests including response to bronchodilators to
discover the maximum respiratory reserve and see if this is
adequate for thoracic surgery

Specific
The following specific tests should be made:
- bronchoscopy, biopsy and brushings for central lesions — to
obtain a definitive histological diagnosis
- percutaneous needle biopsy if the mass is peripheral — to
obtain a cytological diagnosis
- tomographs and CT scans (Fig. 122) are often performed,
but they are expensive and add little to the plain chest X-ray
as far as the diagnosis of a mass is concerned. CT scans are
useful, however, in assessing mediastinal or contralateral
metastases when staging patients for surgery or
chemotherapy if spread is not already obvious on a plain
X-ray.

*Searching for metastases — order of preference for
investigations*

	CT Scan	Radioisotope scan	Ultrasound
Brain	1	2	—
Liver	3	2	1
Bone	—	1*	—
Adrenal	2	—	1

* In conjunction with changes on plain X-ray

Therapy

Surgery
Surgery provides the best hope of a cure for lung cancer. 25%
of patients with operable tumours live for 5 years or more. The
factors which affect operability are described in the following
paragraphs.

Age. Mortality rises progressively with age. Those people aged
over 70 do not tolerate pneumonectomy well.

Local invasion. Recurrent laryngeal nerve palsies, persistent

5.10 Carcinoma of the bronchus

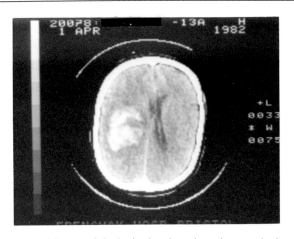

Fig. 122 *CT scan of the brain showing a large intracerebral tumour, a secondary from a bronchial carcinoma.*

pleural effusions, Horner's syndrome, brachial plexus involvement or tumour within 2 cm of carina on the left all preclude surgery. Phrenic nerve palsies preclude surgery unless the left nerve is invaded as it crosses the pericardium where it can be resected.

Non metastatic manifestations. These do not preclude surgery — indeed they may improve following excision of the primary.

Distant metastases. Surgery is contraindicated if there are brain, liver, bone, skin or distant lymph node metastases. This applies also with metastases in the mediastinal lymph nodes — shown either on CT scan or by mediastinoscopy (the latter is more reliable because histology is obtained).

Lung function. It is difficult to generalize, each patient must be taken on his own merits, but guidelines are:
- $FEV_1 > 1.0$ l essential to contemplate any surgical therapy
- $FEV_1 > 60\%$ of predicted — no problems
- $FEV_1 < 40\%$ of predicted — severe post-operative dyspnoea and high peri-operative mortality
- elevated Pa_{CO_2} — contraindication to surgery

233

5.0 Some important diseases

5.10 Carcinoma of the bronchus

Surgical resection. Effects of surgical resections for cancer on
lung function:
- lobectomy leads to a 15% loss of the overall lung volume
  (total lung capacity, TLC) measured with the tumour *in situ*
- pneumonectomy leads to a 30% loss in TLC

Radiotherapy
'Curative' doses of radiotherapy are given to localized
otherwise operable tumours in patients with inadequate
respiratory reserve. Palliative radiotherapy is helpful for:
- troublesome haemoptysis
- painful primary or secondary lesions
- intracerebral secondaries (in addition to dexamethasone and
  phenytoin)
- superior vena caval obstruction
- relieving symptomatic bronchial obstruction

Chemotherapy
Small (oat) cell tumours are sensitive to chemotherapy. This
may be given alone or as an adjuvant either to surgery (rarely
possible) or radiotherapy. Regimens are constantly changing,
but current regimens include combination of
cyclophosphamide, vincristine and VP_{16}. Patients are best
referred to specialized centres for commencement of this
therapy.

Terminal care

Many patients with lung cancer present with advanced
metastatic disease and an accordingly poor prognosis. The
layman's concept of terminal cancer is often one of unabated
pain and suffering. However, with good medical and nursing
management, the patient's quality of life can be maintained
right up to death. The following sections detail some of the
common problems.

Pain
It is useful to find the cause of pain so that specific therapy as
well as non-specific analgesia can be given.

Metastases — specific analgesia. This can be given to relieve
pain in:
- bone — local prostaglandin secretion stimulates nerve

234

endings, thus non-steroidal anti-inflammatory agents are the drugs of choice, such as aspirin 600 mg 4-hourly or indomethacin 50 mg 4-hourly. Local radiotherapy is also helpful
- cerebral — often presenting with headaches and vomiting or fits or focal signs. Dexamethasone 4 mg 6-hourly, is given, reducing slowly to 4–6 mg daily after a week, with cranial irradiation, and prophylactic phenytoin 100 mg 8-hourly to control distressing convulsions.

Non-specific analgesia. Dying patients should be given **regular** analgesia in doses adequate to control their pain. The patient should not wait for the pain to recur before the next dose is given. As life-expectancy is short, drug addiction is not a serious worry. The following drugs are given according to the degree of pain experienced:
- mild pain — aspirin 600 mg or paracetamol 1 g 4-hourly
- moderate pain — soluble aspirin and papaveretum tablets 4-hourly or slow-release morphine tablets (MST) 10 mg 12-hourly initially
- severe pain — oral morphine 5–10 mg 4-hourly or diamorphine 2.5–5.0 mg 4-hourly, or more regularly if the pain demands

These drugs should be given with an anti-emetic, prochlorperazine 5 mg or chlorpromazine 25 mg orally.

If the patient is unable to take oral opiates, half the oral dose may be injected i.m.; alternatively, oxycodone suppositories 30 mg can be given.

Nausea and vomiting

Specific therapy. Look for a treatable cause, such as the following:
- constipation — treat with danthron and poloxane 5–10 ml 12-hourly
- raised intracranial pressure — due to cerebral metastases. Treat with dexamethasone and phenytoin together with radiotherapy if indicated
- hypercalcaemia — treat with oral prednisone 40 mg daily with a high fluid intake and oral phosphate
- hiccoughs — due to phrenic nerve invasion or diaphragmatic

235

irritation. Treat with chlorpromazine 25 mg or
metoclopramide 10 mg

Non-specific anti-emetics. The following are examples:
- phenothiazines — chlorpromazine 25 mg orally or injected or
  prochlorperazine 5 mg orally or injected
- metoclopramide 10 mg orally or injected
- antihistamines — cyclizine 50 mg orally or injected

Cough
Codeine linctus or opiates given for pain relief are normally very
successful in suppressing irritating coughs. With intractable
coughs nebulized bupivicaine may be tried.

Shortness of breath
The cause of the shortness of breath must be found and
treated, e.g. aspirate a pleural effusion, give bronchodilators for
coexistent airways obstruction, or diuretics for heart failure,
give radiotherapy if a lobe is collapsed. Give dexamethasone
(8–12 mg daily initially) for lymphangitis carcinomatosis (more
specific chemotherapy may be available, e.g. for breast
cancer). Non-specific treatment includes oxygen therapy and
morphine or diamorphine which reduce the sensation of
breathlessness, probably by a central action.

Anxiety and depression
Most patients are helped more by sympathetic conversation
than by psychotropic drugs. However, certain patients may
benefit from diazepam 5 mg 8-hourly, or chlorpromazine 25 mg
8-hourly. Patients with religious beliefs will be greatly helped by
the clergy.

Hospices
Hospices (homes for the terminally ill) specialize in caring for
cancer patients through the last few months of their lives,
some also run domiciliary units visiting patients in their own
home. In certain areas there are also health visitors and Marie
Curie nurses specializing in the care of the dying. Local social
workers will know what is available. Social workers can also
play an important role in counselling the rest of the family and
offering as much practical and financial assistance as is
possible.

5.0 Some important diseases

5.10 Carcinoma of the bronchus

Patient education in those receiving palliative therapy. Tell the patient's next of kin the diagnosis and prognosis. To the patient give truthful answers to any questions he asks, but give a slightly more favourable prognosis to provide some hope. If the patient has been given adequate opportunity to ask direct questions but does not do so, do not force the diagnosis upon him unless there are specific family or financial reasons which make it essential for him to be told, so that he can 'put his affairs in order'.

Prognosis

The average time from diagnosis to death is approximately 9 months. The overall 5-year survival is only 5%.

Prevention

Tobacco smoking should be actively discouraged. Atmospheric pollution should be reduced to a minimum. Special precautions should be taken to protect employees working with asbestos, chromates, haematite, nickel and arsenic, all of which have been implicated in the causation of lung cancer.

5.11 Other lung tumours

Alveolar cell (bronchiolar) carcinoma

This cell type comprises less than 1% of all lung tumours. It occurs in the same age group as the other lung cancers. The tumour may be multicentre in origin, arising from alveolar cells and growing throughout alveolar airspaces rather than invading the lung.

Clinical features
- Breathlessness
- Copious watery sputum
- Haemoptysis
- Hypoxic respiratory failure
- Often no abnormal chest signs until very late
- Occasionally finger clubbing

5.0 Some important diseases

5.11   Other lung tumours

Investigations
- Chest X-ray appearance varies from a solitary lesion to widespread alveolar shadowing
- Sputum cytology is usually positive
- Transbronchial or other lung biopsy is the definitive diagnostic procedure

Therapy
Alveolar cell carcinoma does not respond to chemotherapy or radiotherapy. Surgery offers the only hope of a cure if the disease is sufficiently localized to be resected. Overall prognosis is slightly better than for other lung cancers.

Bronchial adenoma (carcinoid and cylindroma)

Much rarer than bronchial carcinoma, representing about 1% of tumours. There are 2 main types, carcinoid and cylindroma. Although sometimes referred to as benign, they are of low-grade malignant potential and may metastasize.

Clinical presentation
Identical to localized carcinoma, but they appear at a younger age and are unrelated to smoking. Very rarely the carcinoid syndrome occurs, but only with metastatic carcinoid tumours (intermittent cyanotic flushes, wheezing, breathlessness, diarrhoea and valvular heart disease). Carcinoids can, rarely, be the source of ectopic hormone secretion.

Investigations
- Chest X-ray may show a visible mass, but is often normal with central tumours. If bronchial obstruction occurs, there may be lobar collapse
- Sputum cytology is unhelpful
- Flow volume loop will demonstrate the obstruction caused by central tumours
- Bronchoscopy and biopsy is the definitive investigation
- Urine tests show raised 5-hydroxyindoleacetic acid levels with metastatic carcinoid tumour

Therapy
Surgical excision is the treatment of choice wherever possible. Radiotherapy is not very successful but is used if the tumour is

inoperable. Prognosis after surgery is good, better for carcinoid tumours than cylindroma.

Hamartoma

A very uncommon benign tumour. Often slightly lobulated with a few specks of calcification visible on X-ray tomography. The diagnosis is usually made after an asymptomatic, well-defined, peripheral lung lesion has been resected in order to exclude a malignant neoplasm.

5.12   Pulmonary embolism

Causes

Pulmonary emboli usually arise from a venous thrombosis in the deep veins of either the pelvis or the legs. Portions of these blood clots break off and are carried through the right side of the heart out into the pulmonary circulation, causing a varying degree of circulatory disturbance depending upon the number, size and distribution of the emboli. Small emboli may be asymptomatic; large ones can be (and often are) fatal. Large emboli may cause pulmonary infarction (Fig. 123), although this happens rarely because of the lung's dual blood supply (pulmonary and bronchial). Pulmonary emboli are found in up to 25% of all patients at post-mortem.

Clinical features

Massive emboli
Massive emboli present acutely with a life-threatening illness characterized by:
- acute severe breathlessness
- sudden central chest discomfort
- cyanosis
- tachycardia
- hypotension
- elevated jugular venous pressure
- sudden death may occur

Smaller emboli
Smaller emboli present as non life-threatening acute illness with

239

5.12 Pulmonary embolism

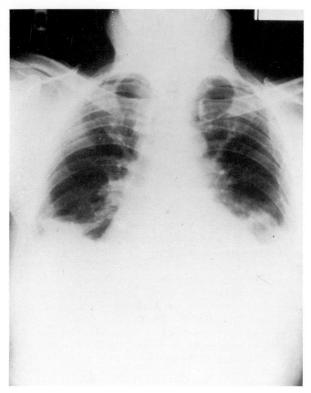

Fig. 123 *Multiple pulmonary infarcts. Note the wedge-shaped shadows at the right base.*

some of these features:
- pleuritic chest pain
- haemoptysis
- breathlessness
- pyrexia
- pleural friction rub
- signs of consolidation

In both groups of patients there are often the signs of peripheral deep vein thrombosis.

5.0 Some important diseases

5.12 Pulmonary embolism

Investigations

These can be divided into direct investigations, searching for evidence of embolism, and indirect, searching for its source.

Direct investigations
- Chest X-ray PA and lateral — this is usually normal in acute episodes, but may show reduced vascular markings. Later, wedge-shaped shadows may be evident with pulmonary infarction
- ECG — in the minority of cases (about 15%) the 'classical' SI, QIII, TIII, pattern is seen (Fig. 124)
- Blood gases — there is hypoxia due to *V/Q* mismatch and hypocapnia due to hyperventilation
- Ventilation/perfusion lung scans — multiple defects on a perfusion scan not matched by a ventilatory defect are diagnostically helpful (Figs 125–7)
- Pulmonary angiogram — the only definitive test, but it is invasive and not without hazard (Fig. 128)

Indirect investigations
- Venography — the best way to demonstrate clots in deep

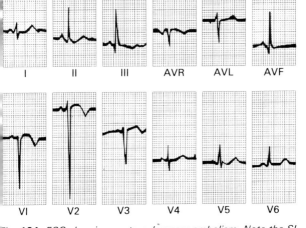

Fig. 124 *ECG showing acute pulmonary embolism. Note the SI QIII TIII pattern together with the inverted T waves in the right chest leads V1 V2.*

5.0 Some important diseases

5.12 Pulmonary embolism

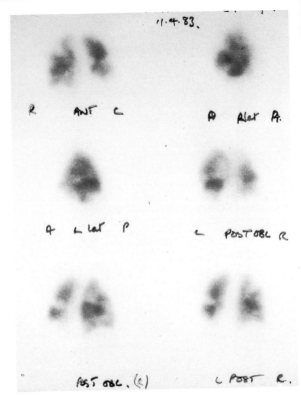

Fig. 125 *Perfusion radioisotope lung scan showing multiple perfusion defects compatible with pulmonary emboli.*

veins of the leg and pelvis, but it is often painful (Fig. 129)
- Ultrasound (Doppler) gives a large number of false negatives both in the calves and pelvic veins.
- I^{125} fibrinogen scanning is of limited use because clots within the abdomen are not demonstrated

Prevention

Awareness of the risk factors concerning deep venous thrombosis enables some, but not all, of them to be avoided:

5.12 Pulmonary embolism

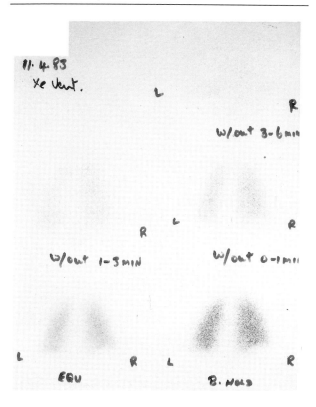

Fig. 126 *Normal ventilation scan of the same patient confirming the perfusion defects to be due to emboli.*

- prolonged sitting, e.g. long air flights
- prolonged bed rest in hospital — hemiplegia, congestive cardiac failure, myocardial infarctions, infections
- surgery
- pregnancy
- high oestrogen contraceptive pill
- smoking
- obesity
- malignancy (e.g. pancreas and bronchus)
- dehydration

5.12 Pulmonary embolism

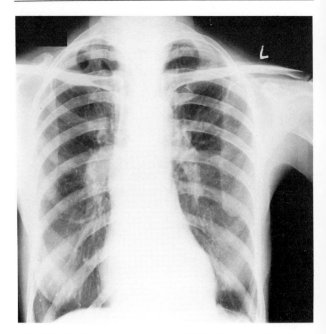

Fig. 127 *Multiple pulmonary emboli. Note the loss of vessel markings particularly in the right mid-zone.*

Patients in bed or anyone on long journeys should be encouraged to move their legs frequently. Prophylactic low-dose calcium heparin 5000 units subcutaneously 8-hourly until the patient is fully ambulant, is often given routinely pre- and post-operatively and in coronary care units.

Therapy

Massive life-threatening pulmonary embolism — emergency resuscitation

1. Perform external cardiac massage.
2. Intubate with an endotracheal tube and ventilate with high oxygen concentration.
3. Analgesia — morphine 10 mg i.m.
4. Anticoagulation — heparin 10 000 units i.v. stat. and

5.12 Pulmonary embolism

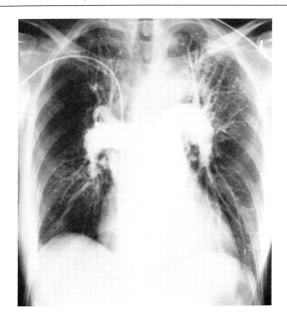

Fig. 128 *Pulmonary angiogram of the same patient confirming the occlusion of many major pulmonary vessels due to emboli.*

10 000 units 6-hourly. Warfarin commenced after 14 days.
5. Streptokinase — via a central catheter directly into the pulmonary artery. 600 000 units in the first ½ hour, then 100 000 units hourly for 72 hours. Hydrocortisone 200 mg 6-hourly is given as prophylaxis against allergic reactions.
   Contraindications to streptokinase therapy are:
   • bleeding disorders
   • peptic ulcers
   • hypertension
   • recent surgery
   • previous cerebrovascular haemorrhage
6. Surgical embolectomy under cardiopulmonary bypass. This is reserved for critically ill patients who show no signs of improvement or who remain very ill in spite of medical therapy. If an emergency pulmonary angiogram shows a reduction of pulmonary perfusion by 75% or more, embolectomy is indicated.

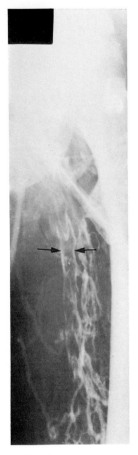

Fig. 129 *Venogram showing extensive venous thrombosis in the left femoral vein. Note the thrombus outlined by contrast running circumferentially.*

5.0 Some important diseases

5.12 Pulmonary embolism

Non-life-threatening pulmonary embolism
In this situation, the following should be implemented:
1. 60% oxygen via a mask.
2. Analgesia — morphine 10 mg i.m.
3. Heparin 10 000 units i.v. 6-hourly for 7 days, commence oral warfarin with dose adjusted according to prothrombin time (or thrombotest) — continued for 3 months.
4. If investigations show a fresh clot in the deep pelvic veins which is likely to re-embolize, surgical procedures such as insertion of an 'umbrella' into or plication of the inferior vena cava may be considered.
5. Clinically it is often difficult to differentiate between pneumonia and a pulmonary embolism. Pulmonary infarcts often become infected. Thus, broad-spectrum antibiotics are often given.

Recurrent thrombo-embolism

There is a small group of patients, often middle-aged women, who have recurrent 'asymptomatic' pulmonary emboli over several years who eventually present with:
- increasing breathlessness
- right heart failure — due to pulmonary hypertension
- hypoxia — at first only on exercise

These patients require life-time anticoagulation with warfarin (any known precipitating factors should be avoided). Heart failure is treated by digoxin and diuretics. Oxygen provides symptomatic relief in the later stages.

5.13 Sarcoidosis

Causes

Sarcoidosis is a multi-system disease of unknown aetiology occurring mainly in the third or fourth decades of life, which is characterized by the presence of non-caseating epithelioid granulomata. Present theories include those of infection with 'L' forms of mycobacteria or other transmissible agents.

5.0 Some important diseases

5.13 Sarcoidosis

Clinical features

The presenting features of sarcoidosis will depend upon which system is primarily affected.

Pulmonary system
The commonest presentation of sarcoidosis in the pulmonary system is through a routine chest X-ray (e.g. mass miniature or pre-employment), or from an X-ray performed because of a minimal 'flu-like' illness. The usual chest X-ray changes are bilateral hilar lymphadenopathy (Stage I; Fig. 130). (Unilateral adenopathy is unusual.) Less often, the hilar adenopathy is associated with parenchymal lung infiltration (Stage II; Fig. 131). Even rarer, is parenchymal lung infiltration or fibrosis alone (Stage III). Parenchymal lung disease may present with cough and shortness of breath. There are often no chest signs. Infiltration and fibrosis may give rise to fine inspiratory crepitations which are usually bilateral.

Skin
• Erythema nodosum is common and is often associated with

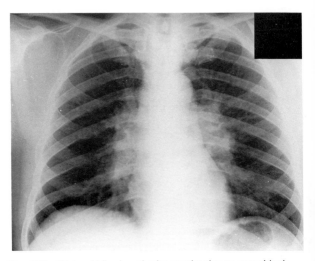

Fig. 130 *Bilateral hilar lymphadenopathy due to sarcoidosis — stage 1.*

5.13 Sarcoidosis

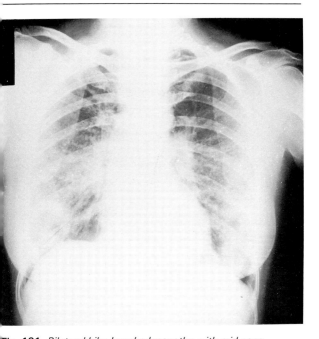

Fig. 131 *Bilateral hilar lymphadenopathy with mid-zone interstitial infiltration — stage 2 sarcoidosis.*

fever, hilar adenopathy and arthralgia (Fig. 132). Other common causes of erythema nodosum are streptococcal infection, drugs, e.g. sulphonamides and the contraceptive pill, and tuberculosis
* Lupus pernio (Fig. 133)
* Localized skin infiltration — may be plaques (Fig. 134), papules or nodules

Eyes
Sarcoidosis affects the eyes through uveitis. Acute iritis is common and presents with painful red eye with impairment of vision. Slit lamp examination should be made in all patients. The lachrymal glands may be enlarged — either alone or in conjunction with the salivary glands (Heerfordt's syndrome; Fig. 135).

5.13 Sarcoidosis

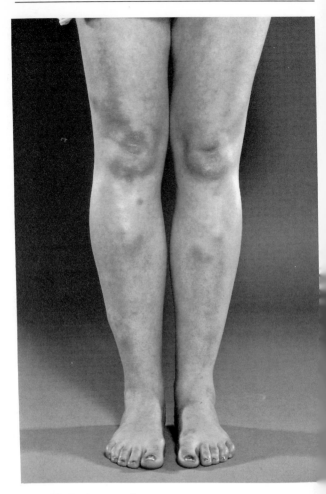

Fig. 132 *Erythema nodosum.*

5.13 Sarcoidosis

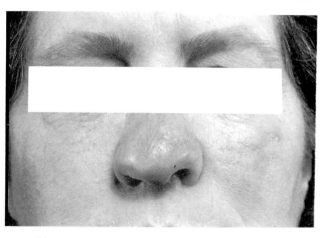

Fig. 133 *Lupus pernio.*

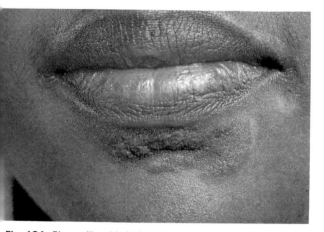

Fig. 134 *Plaque-like skin lesion due to sarcoidosis.*

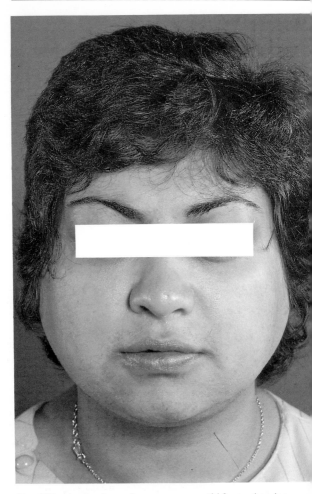

Fig. 135 *Heerfordt syndrome, uveoparotid fever showing enlargement of the salivary and lachrymal glands.*

5.0 Some important diseases

5.13 Sarcoidosis

Reticuloendothelial system
- Lymphadenopathy — commonly cervical but may affect any nodes
- Hepatosplenomegaly — splenomegaly is usually asymptomatic but there can be pain or a dragging feeling from a very large spleen. Hypersplenism is rare. Hepatomegaly is also usually asymptomatic but may, rarely, be associated with pain or jaundice and weight loss

Skeletal and neuromuscular systems
- Arthralgia — primarily affecting the large peripheral joints: wrists, elbows, ankles and knees. Often associated with erythema nodosum, hilar adenopathy and fever
- Bone disease — cysts develop in the phalanges. They have a characteristic 'punched-out' appearance on X-ray (Fig. 136)
- Bell's palsy — lower motor neurone VII cranial nerve palsy (Fig. 137)
- Peripheral neuropathy — mixed sensorimotor
- Intracerebral sarcoid — sarcoid deposits acting like a space-occupying lesion

Metabolic and endocrine systems
- Hypercalcaemia or hypercalciuria — these are usually

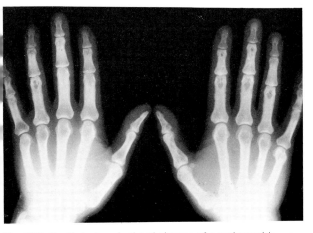

Fig. 136 *Cystic lesions in the phalanges of a patient with sarcoidosis.*

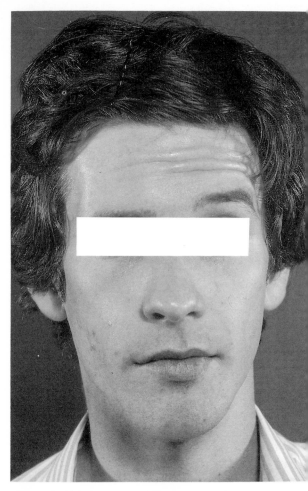

Fig. 137 *Right lower motor neurone seventh cranial nerve palsy due to sarcoidosis. Note the loss of facial expression over the forehead as well as the weakness of the rest of the right side of the face.*

asymptomatic but may lead to nephrocalcinosis and renal failure. Increased levels of 1,25 dihydroxycholecalciferol are found. Hypercalciuria (6%) is more common than hypercalcaemia (2%)

- Diabetes insipidus — sarcoid deposits may occur in the posterior pituitary gland impairing ADH secretion

Cardiac system

- Cor pulmonale due to pulmonary hypertension developing from pulmonary fibrosis (rare)
- Cardiomyopathy due to sarcoid deposition in the heart muscle presenting as arrhythmias, congestive cardiac failure or sudden death (even rarer)

Investigations

Radiology

- Chest X-ray — the most frequent abnormalities are those of bilateral hilar and mediastinal lymphadenopathy with or without mid-zone parenchymal infiltration or fibrosis
- Plain abdominal X-ray — check for nephrocalcinosis or renal calculi (complications of hypercalciuria), or hepatosplenomegaly

Physiology

- Lung function tests — spirometry and gas transfer are normal except with infiltration or fibrosis when first the gas transfer and then the lung volumes deteriorate

Bacteriology

- Sputum — a very careful search must be made on at least 3 occasions to exclude the presence of mycobacterium tuberculosis
- Biopsy specimens — the same is true

Haematology

- Blood count — there is often a lymphopenia (T-lymphocytes become sequestered in the granuloma)
- ESR — non-specifically elevated in active disease

Biochemistry

- Liver function tests — elevated alkaline phosphatase is common with liver granuloma

5.0 Some important diseases

5.13 Sarcoidosis

- Serum calcium and 24-hour urinary calcium measurements
- Urea and electrolytes ⎫ To check renal function (may
- Creatinine clearance ⎬ be impaired due to hypercalciuria
  ⎭ or granulomata in the kidney
- Serum angiotension converting enzyme (SACE) — the elevation of this enzyme is related to the activity of the sarcoidosis, hence it may be used to monitor disease activity. Occasionally it is elevated in other granulomatous conditions such as leprosy and Gaucher's disease. Steroid therapy suppresses the level of SACE. ACE is produced bo by activated monocytes within granulomata and by the pulmonary capillary endothelial cells

Immunology
- Serum immune complexes are frequently present particular with erythema nodosum and arthralgia
- Serum immunoglobulins, IgG, IgM and IgA, are all usually non-specifically elevated
- Delayed hypersensitivity skin reactions, tuberculin, candida mumps and dinitrochlorobenzene (DNCB) skin tests, are usually negative in active disease. These recover when the disease has resolved. In-vitro lymphocyte transformation to plant lectins such as PHA and ConA is also depressed in active disease.

Radioisotope gallium scans (Fig. 138)
Active granuloma accumulate gallium-67 after it is injected. Scans of the chest taken 2–3 days afterwards give an idea of the distribution of the disease activity. However, gallium may also be taken up by lymphoma, tuberculosis and any active alveolitis (e.g. fibrosing alveolitis) and thus its use is limited to assessing the disease activity rather than diagnosis.

Histology
None of the tests listed previously are diagnostic of sarcoidosis, hence in all cases histology should be obtained.

Kveim skin test. If sarcoidosis is strongly suspected with no suspicion of lymphoma or TB, it is reasonable to wait for the results of a Kveim skin test to confirm the diagnosis. The mai disadvantage of this test (apart from a false negative in 20–30%) is that it takes 4–6 weeks to develop before a biop is performed.

5.13 Sarcoidosis

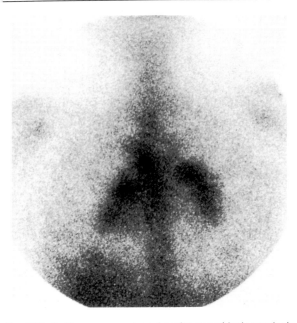

Fig. 138 *Gallium scan — stage 1 active sarcoidosis uptake in hilar nodes.*

Tissue biopsy. A histological diagnosis may be obtained from many sites depending upon the clinical presentation. The commonest biopsy sites are:

- lung — bronchial or transbronchial biopsy together with bronchoalveolar lavage. Biopsy is positive in up to 80% of patients. The alveolar lavage in acute active parenchymal disease contains a high percentage (>25%) of lymphocytes (mostly activated helper T-cells). The lymphocyte count can be used to monitor disease activity by repeated lavage over several months
- lymph nodes — cervical, scalene or mediastinal (from mediastinoscopy)
- liver
- skin nodules
- lachrymal gland

5.13 Sarcoidosis

If granulomata are found in the biopsy, a careful search must be made for mycobacteria to exclude tuberculosis.

Therapy

Most patients with sarcoidosis need careful observation with no active therapy because the disease usually resolves spontaneously. At each visit, the patient should be interviewed, examined and a chest X-ray and lung function tests (spirometry and gas transfer) should be performed. Serum angiotensin converting enzyme should be estimated and calcium status (blood and urine) should be checked regularly. Active therapy, if indicated, is usually with oral corticosteroids

Indications for steroid therapy
- Pulmonary disease — parenchymal disease which is either symptomatic (breathlessness), progressive or failing to clear spontaneously after 6 months observation (judged by chest X-ray or lung function testing). The object is to prevent permanent fibrosis
- Uveitis always requires therapy — steroid eyedrops initially
- Persistent hypercalcaemia or hypercalciuria readily respond to steroids and should be treated to avoid renal damage
- Bell's palsy often responds to high doses of steroids
- Intracranial deposits are often unresponsive, but high-dose steroids should be tried (e.g. prednisone 80 mg/day)
- Lupus pernio and other skin diseases require local rather than systemic therapy. They should be treated for cosmetic reasons
- Parotid and lachrymal enlargement — also mainly for cosmetic reasons
- Myocardial disease to avoid arrhythmias and cardiac failure

Dosage of steroids
Other than for intracranial deposits the starting dose of steroid is prednisone 30 mg/day reducing to a maintenance dose of around 10 mg/day after initial response. The initial course is for 6 months. Chronic disease often needs 5–10 mg/day and may recur when lower doses are reached. Treatment may be lifelong.

5.0 Some important diseases

5.13 Sarcoidosis

Prognosis

In the vast majority of patients sarcoidosis is a trivial self-limiting disease. In a very few, especially those with intracranial or myocardial involvement, it can be rapidly fatal. Bilateral hilar lymphadenopathy takes an average of 8 months to regress. Spontaneous resolution occurring within 1 year in 80% and within 2 years in 90% of patients. With hilar adenopathy and parenchymal shadows, 50% of patients clear spontaneously, and a further 30% with steroid therapy. In Stage III disease (parenchymal shadowing alone) the outlook is worse with only 40% of patients remitting even with steroid therapy. If pulmonary sarcoidosis does not regress, it can lead to pulmonary fibrosis and cor pulmonale due to pulmonary hypertension.

5.14 Industrial lung disease

Coal worker's pneumoconiosis

This is the commonest dust disease in the UK. Several hundred new cases are registered each year. Considerable exposure over 15–20 years is usually needed. The condition is caused by alveolar deposition of very small (1–3 μm) coal dust particles. These are ingested by macrophages which die in the process releasing their harmful enzymes leading to a local fibrotic process. Coal dust is less fibrogenic than silica.

Clinical features

Simple pneumoconiosis is due to the lungs gradually filling with coal dust, but causing little fibrosis. Its features are:

- asymptomatic
- chest X-ray shows multiple opacities, particularly in upper zones. The opacities vary in size: punctiform (up to 1.5 mm); miliary (1.5–3.0 mm), or nodular (3–10 mm)
- coexisting chronic bronchitis is common

Complicated pneumoconiosis is due to progressive massive fibrosis (PMF; Fig. 139), featuring:

- breathlessness
- fibrotic masses several centimetres in diameter in the upper lobes

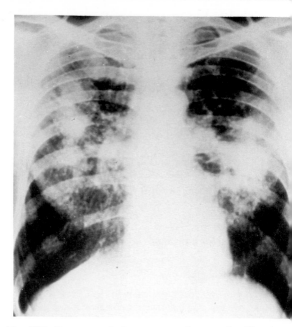

Fig. 139 *Pneumoconiosis — progressive massive fibrosis, confluent interstitial shadowing giving rise to mass-like lesio*

- bronchiectasis
- cor pulmonale may eventually develop
- finger clubbing does *not* occur

Caplan's syndrome
- Rheumatoid arthritis
- Pneumoconiosis
- Peripheral round pulmonary rheumatoid nodules (0.5–5.0 cm) which may cavitate

Therapy
- Remove from exposure to coal dust
- Treat coexisting chronic bronchitis
- Claim compensation through the UK Industrial Injuries Act that the patient can be assessed by a Pneumoconiosis Par

5.0 Some important diseases

5.14 Industrial lung disease

who categorize the severity of the disease referring to standard X-rays (see Table 11)

Table 11 Categories of coal worker's pneumoconiosis assessed by chest X-ray changes.

Category	Small, rounded lung opacities	Lung markings
0	absent	normal
1	few	normal
2	numerous	still visible
3	very numerous	partly or totally obscured

Silicosis

Inhaled silica is a very fibrogenic material. Exposure occurs in:
- metal mining (gold, tin, copper)
- quarrying of granite, sandstone and slate
- sandblasting
- boiler scaling
- pottery and ceramic manufacture

The silica particles are toxic to the alveolar macrophages which ingest them. The macrophages then release their enzymes leading to pulmonary inflammation and fibrosis.

Clinical features
- Progressive shortness of breath
- Restrictive ventilatory defect
  ($\downarrow$ FEV$_1$, $\downarrow$ FVC, $\uparrow$ or normal FEV$_1$/FVC%, $\downarrow$ gas transfer (DLCO))
- Diffuse miliary or nodular pattern on X-ray — mainly upper and mid zones. The hilar lymph glands may show eggshell calcification
- Increased incidence of tuberculosis

Therapy
- Removal from exposure
- Obtain compensation through the Pneumoconiosis Panel set up under the UK Industrial Injuries Act

5.0 Some important diseases

5.14 Industrial lung disease

Asbestos-related disease

Asbestos consists of the silicates of iron, magnesium, nickel calcium and aluminium.

Types of asbestos
- Chrysotile — coiled fibres, 'white'
- Crocidolite — straight fibres, 'blue'
- Anthophyllite
- Amosite

Uses
- Fireproofing
- Brake linings
- Cement
- Tiles
- Tyres
- Roofing felt
- Pipe lagging
- Electric wire insulation

Asbestosis

Asbestosis is pulmonary fibrosis related to the amount of asbestos exposure. This condition is caused through local irritation by asbestos fibres which are cleared very slowly from the alveoli. The clinical features are those of other fibrotic lung diseases.

Pleural plaques (Fig. 140)

Asbestos fibres have a high penetration and so cause pleural irritation. This may occur together with, or independently of, asbestosis. With pleural plaques the risk of carcinoma of the bronchus is doubled. Plaques are often bilateral and very numerous.

Lung cancer

The incidence of lung cancer in patients with asbestosis is estimated at 20%. There is a synergism with cigarette smoking.

262

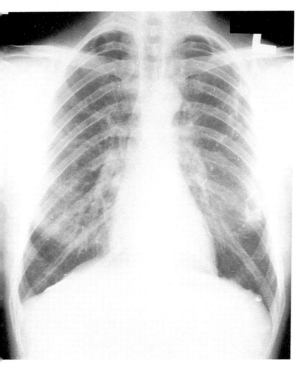

Fig. 140 *Calcification of the diaphragmatic pleura together with left pleural plaques due to asbestos exposure.*

Mesothelioma (Fig. 141)

Only minimal asbestos exposure is needed to develop a mesothelioma. Crocidolite, in particular, is implicated since its alveolar penetration is 6 times that of chrysotile due to its fibre shape. The latent period between the exposure and tumour development is about 40 years. The association with pleural plaques is still uncertain.

Clinical features of mesothelioma
There is often a coexisting (blood-stained) pleural effusion. The commonest symptoms are those of dyspnoea and chest pain

263

5.14 Industrial lung disease

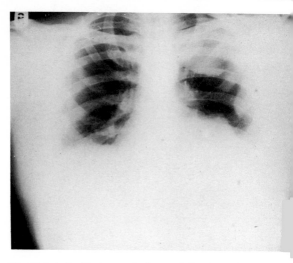

Fig. 141 *Left-sided mesothelioma of the pleura due to asbestos exposure.*

together with weight loss. The signs are those of pleural thickening and fluid. Other symptoms and signs may be caus~~ed~~ by spread.

Local. Mesothelioma may spread locally to:
- heart and pericardium — pain, atrial fibrillation and heart failure
- contralateral pleura — pain and breathlessness
- chest wall — pain
- chest scars — may grow through thoracotomy or biopsy scars

Distant. In particular there may be spread to:
- mediastinal and hilar lymph nodes
- liver
- lung
- bone

These may all coexist with a peritoneal mesothelioma which usually presents with abdominal pain and obstruction.

5.0 Some important diseases

5.14 Industrial lung disease

Investigation
The diagnosis is made on histology after seeing a chest X-ray.
Pleural biopsy using an Abram's needle often provides an
inadequate specimen, thus open pleural biopsy is usually
required. However, a definitive diagnosis is often not made
until post-mortem. There are a wide range of histological
appearances:

- tubopapillary
- mixed
- sarcomatous
- undifferentiated polygonal

More than one type may be present in the same tumour.

Therapy
Surgery, radiotherapy and chemotherapy all have little to offer.
Prognosis is 1–2 years from diagnosis.

Compensation

Asbestosis, severe pleural disease (if causing a disability) and
mesothelioma are financially compensatible diseases under the
UK Industrial Injuries Act. A pneumoconiosis medical panel can
award a pension to the patient or his family. The coroner must
be informed if a patient is suspected of dying from an asbestos-
related disease.

5.15 Cryptogenic fibrosing alveolitis

Causes

The interstitium of the lung may become fibrosed as the end
result of the alveolitis associated with numerous well-
recognized diseases (see Table 12). When no such associated
condition exists the term cryptogenic fibrosing alveolitis is
applied. The role of immune complexes in the causation of
cryptogenic fibrosing alveolitis is currently under investigation.

Clinical features

The patient presents with a dry cough and progressive
shortness of breath — initially on exertion, then at rest. The
diagnosis is made as follows.

5.0 Some important diseases

5.15 Cryptogenic fibrosing alveolitis

Table 12 Causes of diffuse pulmonary fibrosis to be excluded before diagnosing cryptogenic fibrosing alveolities.

- industrial exposure — coal miner's pneumoconiosis
  silicosis
  asbestosis
  berylliosis
- sarcoidosis
- extrinsic allergic alveolitis — bird fancier's lung
  farmer's lung
- chronic pulmonary oedema — mitral stenosis
- connective tissue disorders — rheumatoid arthritis
  SLE
  scleroderma
- radiotherapy
- drugs — gold
  cyclophosphamide
  bleomycin
  nitrofurantoin
  sulphasalazine
  busulphan
  hexamethonium
- severe organized pneumonias
- histiocytosis X

Lymphangitis carcinomatosis also frequently comes into the differential diagnosis of a breathless patient with diffuse interstitial shadowing on X-ray, but clearly the lung changes in this case are not those of fibrosis

Obligatory for the diagnosis
- Widespread radiographic shadows — bilateral, reticular, mainly lower zones (Fig. 142). Honeycombing may occur in advanced disease. Pleural disease is rare
- All known extrinsic causes excluded
- Compatible histology
- If no histology is available, widespread crepitations present — usually end inspiratory

Supportive of the diagnosis
- Finger clubbing (very rarely hypertrophic pulmonary osteoarthropathy may also occur)
- Restrictive ventilatory defect

266

5.15 Cryptogenic fibrosing alveolitis

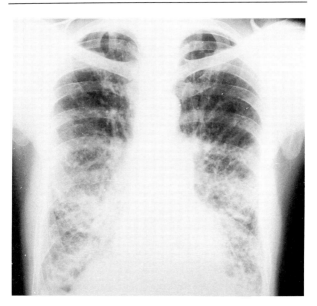

Fig. 142 *Cryptogenic fibrosing alveolitis. Note the bilateral mainly basal interstitial reticulonodular shadowing.*

Investigations

- Chest X-ray — loss of lung volume as well as the changes mentioned above
- Lung function tests — a restrictive defect with relative preservation of peak flow rate. Low FEV_1 and FVC with normal or increased FEV_1/FVC% — reduced TLC, reduced gas transfer. Low compliance, i.e. small, stiff lungs
- Blood gases — hypoxia, initially only on exertion then later even at rest (widened alveolar–arterial oxygen gradient due to *V/Q* mismatch). Hypocapnia due to hyperventilation
- Elevated ESR — non-specific
- Immunological tests — ANF positive 30%, rheumatoid factor positive 10%, immune complexes often detected, complement levels normal
- Lung biopsy — it is always advisable to have a histological diagnosis. Transbronchial biopsy is the safest technique, but has the disadvantage of providing small samples. For this

5.0   Some important diseases

5.15   Cryptogenic fibrosing alveolitis

reason, and because the disease is not always uniform throughout the lung, open lung biopsy is preferred. However the patient must be fit enough and the extra information obtained from larger biopsies must be likely to alter the management. A trephine drill biopsy provides a compromise between the 2 methods but should only be done by a very skilled operator.

Histology shows 2 main abnormalities, a relative neutrophili in the alveolar spaces with an increase in cellular thickening and fibrous material in alveolar walls, 2 main patterns are recognized.

Usual Interstitial Pneumonia (UIP) is the commoner, consisting of a fibrocellular infiltrate of the alveolar walls.

Desquamative Interstitial Pneumonia (DIP) — there is also desquamation of macrophages and type II pneumocytes.
- Bronchoalveolar lavage — in patients with adequate respiratory reserve ($FEV_1 > 1.0$ l, $PaO_2 > 50$ mmHg (6.5 kPa)) performed at the same time as transbronchial biopsy. This technique is of little diagnostic value, but it ma provide a method of assessing the activity of the alveolitis. There is an increase in the total cell yield with a relative increase in neutrophils in CFA
- Gallium-67 scanning will also demonstrate the activity of th alveolitis but is not a diagnostic test

Complications

- Progressive type I (hypoxic) respiratory failure
- Increased risk of lung cancer

Therapy

Corticosteroid therapy is tried in virtually all cases. It is sometimes successful, and is most likely to work in the following instances:
- young patients who are not very breathless
- active alveolitis on bronchoalveolar lavage, or gallium scan
- DIP histology
- little fibrosis already present

5.0 Some important diseases

5.15 Cryptogenic fibrosing alveolitis

Prednisone 60 mg is given daily for 4 weeks, then gradually tailed down to 10 mg daily if there is a response. If there is no response, cyclophosphamide 1.5 mg/kg daily is given. The value of other drugs such as penicillamine is unproven.

Assessment of response
As well as subjective symptomatic improvement it is important to have objective improvement, hence a chest X-ray and lung function tests are performed at each visit. Recently, the alveolitis has begun to be assessed by a combination of repeated bronchoalveolar lavages and gallium scans. With successful therapy the percentage of neutrophils in the lavage falls and the gallium scan becomes 'cold'.

Prognosis

Not all patients respond to therapy. The average time between diagnosis and death varies between 1 and 30 years with a mean of 6 years. In general, the longer the length of history on presentation the better the prognosis. DIP has a better prognosis than UIP.

5.16 Extrinsic allergic alveolitis

Causes (see Table 13)

In sensitized individuals, the inhalation and alveolar deposition of small organic particles (1–5 μm) leads to a local type III immune response mediated by antigen–antibody complexes which activate the complement cascade. In the acute phase, the alveoli are infiltrated with acute inflammatory cells — lymphocytes, plasma cells and neutrophils together with fibrin deposition. Later, with continued exposure, granuloma formation and obliterative bronchiolitis occurs.

Clinical features

Acute episodes
4–6 hours after antigen exposure:
- fever
- rigors
- myalgia

5.0 Some important diseases

5.16 Extrinsic allergic alveolitis

Table 13 Some examples of extrinsic allergic alveolitis.

Disease	Antigen	Source
Farmer's lung	*Micropolyspora faeni* *Thermoactinomyces vulgaris*	Mouldy hay
Bird fancier's lung } Pigeon fancier's lung }	Serum protein in bird droppings	Bird droppings — budgerigar or pigeon
Malt worker's lung	*Aspergillus clavatus*	Mouldy barley
Humidifier fever	Thermophilic actinomyces	Air conditioners Humidifiers
Mushroom worker's lung	*M. faeni* *T. vulgaris*	Mushroom compost
Bagassosis	*T. sacchari*	Mouldy bagasse (sugar cane)

- breathlessness **without wheeze**
- dry cough
- ubiquitous crepitations

Complications with chronic exposure
Pulmonary fibrosis and eventually pulmonary hypertension occur causing:
- increasing breathlessness
- weight loss
- respiratory failure — type I (hypoxic)
- cor pulmonale

Investigations

Chest X-ray
- Acute phase — mottling or consolidation in the mid-zones. Hilar adenopathy is very rare
- With repeated attacks there is fibrosis, particularly of the upper lobe, leading eventually to honeycomb lung

Pulmonary function
This shows a restrictive defect ($\downarrow$TLC, $\downarrow$FVC, $\downarrow$FEV$_1$ normal or $\uparrow$FEV$_1$/FVC%) with low gas transfer (DLCO) in acute attacks. Initially the changes are reversed by removal from the antigen but with repeated exposure the lung function abnormalities persist.

5.0 Some important diseases

5.16 Extrinsic allergic alveolitis

Blood
Eosinophilia does *not* occur.

Blood gases
Hypoxia and low $Paco_2$ in attacks.

Serum precipitins
These may be sought to specific antigens (see Table 13). Their presence is not diagnostic in that they are also found in some asymptomatic subjects who have been exposed to the same antigens.

Skin tests
There is a positive delayed skin response to specific antigen at 4–6 hours.

Therapy

Acute episodes
- Removal from antigen
- Oxygen 35% or higher concentration
- Intravenous hydrocortisone 200 mg followed by oral prednisone 40–60 mg daily, the daily dose reducing by 10 mg each week once the disease is controlled

Chronic disease
Whenever possible, patients with extrinsic allergic alveolitis should be advised to avoid all exposure to the harmful antigen even if this requires a change of job or giving up their hobby. If this is impossible, they should wear effective masks, such as the Baxter 'Pneu-Seal' or the Racal 'airstream' positive pressure powered respiratory helmet.

Compensation

Farmer's lung and malt worker's lung are both acknowledged occupational diseases under the UK Industrial Injuries Act and a person contracting these diseases in the UK is entitled to Industrial Injuries Benefit.

Prognosis

The outlook for acute attacks is very good. However, after persistent prolonged exposure, pulmonary fibrosis, 'end stage lung' and respiratory failure occur — hence the importance of avoiding antigen exposure as early as possible.

5.17 Aspergillus and lung disease

Types of disease

The aspergillus group of fungi may cause a number of distinct pulmonary diseases. *Aspergillus fumigatus* is the most frequently implicated pathogen.
1. Simple extrinsic asthma — precipitated by spore inhalation.
2. Allergic bronchopulmonary aspergillosis.
3. Aspergilloma — fungal ball in cavities usually from previous tuberculosis.
4. Invasive aspergillosis, e.g. in the immunosuppressed.
5. Extrinsic allergic alveolitis, e.g. malt worker's lung (*Asp. clavatus*).

Investigations

In all the forms of aspergillus lung disease, aspergillus is found in the sputum and precipitating antibodies are found in the serum except in simple extrinsic asthma. Eosinophilia is found only in allergic bronchopulmonary aspergillosis. Positive immediate skin tests to aspergillus are found in all patients with allergic bronchopulmonary aspergillosis and all those with simple asthma as well as 30% of those with an aspergilloma. Late skin tests are typical of patients with allergic bronchopulmonary aspergillosis, but are also found in some patients with an aspergilloma.

Allergic bronchopulmonary aspergillosis (Figs 143–6)

Clinical features
- Asthma
- Eosinophilia — in blood and sputum
- Transient segmental areas of collapse and consolidation on

5.17 Aspergillus and lung disease

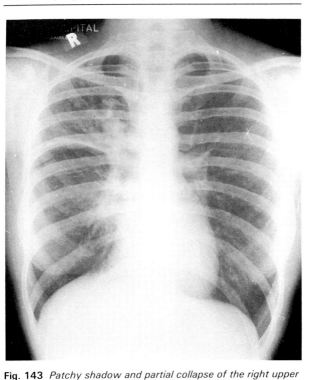

Fig. 143 *Patchy shadow and partial collapse of the right upper lobe due to bronchopulmonary aspergillosis.*

chest X-ray beyond mucus plugs containing aspergillus hyphae — mainly in the upper lobes

Investigations
- Aspergillus in sputum
- Positive immediate and delayed aspergillus skin tests
- Positive serum precipitins for aspergillus

Complications
Proximal bronchiectasis is a complication in areas affected by transient collapse and consolidation.

5.17 Aspergillus and lung disease

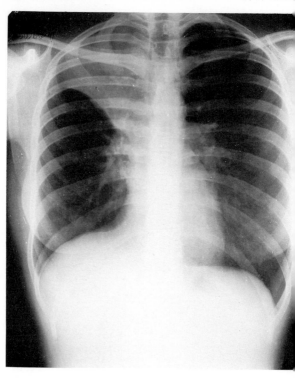

Fig. 144 *The same patient as shown in Fig. 143 — separate episode of right upper lobe collapse/consolidation.*

Therapy
Oral prednisone is given, 30 mg daily until acute attack has settled and then reducing to a maintenance dose of 5–10 mg daily to prevent segmental collapse and later bronchiectasis. Inhaled steroids are ineffective. Routine bronchodilator therapy is given as in other forms of asthma.

Aspergilloma

A fungus ball usually of aspergillus fumigatus may grow with a pre-existing lung cavity. The cavity most commonly being caused by previous tuberculosis (Fig. 147).

5.17 Aspergillus and lung disease

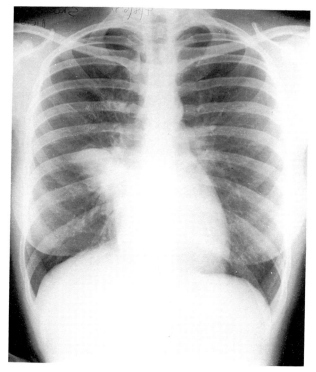

Fig. 145 *The same patient — right hilar mass effect with flare.*

Clinical features

Aspergilloma may be asymptomatic but frequent symptoms include:

* haemoptysis — may be copious
* lethargy
* weight loss

Investigations

* Chest X-ray — opacity within a cavity
* Sputum — mycelia and growth of aspergillus
* Serum precipitins — strongly positive with multiple precipitin lines

275

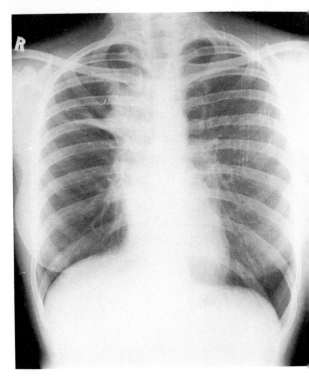

Fig. 146 *The same patient — further episode of right upper lobe collapse/consolidation.*

- Immediate skin test — positive to aspergillus in 30%
- Late skin test to aspergillus — occasionally positive

Therapy
In asymptomatic patients, no therapy is needed, but surgical removal is the treatment of choice for solitary symptomatic lesions. Numerous drug therapies have been tried unsuccessfully.

5.0 Some important diseases

5.17 Aspergillus and lung disease

Extrinsic allergic alveolitis

'Malt worker's lung' is due to sensitivity to *Aspergillus clavatus*. The clinical features and therapy are as for other causes of extrinsic allergic alveolitis. Diagnosis is made from the history of exposure and the presence of serum precipitins to *Asp. clavatus*. If untreated, pulmonary fibrosis eventually occurs. Compensation is payable under the UK Industrial Injuries Act.

Invasive aspergillosis

Aspergillus hyphae may invade lung parenchyma. This occurs in the immunosuppressed, particularly after broad-spectrum antibiotics.

Investigations
- Sputum — fungal hyphae on smear and heavy growth of aspergillus
- Serum precipitins for aspergillus are found
- Chest X-ray — area of consolidation sometimes with abscess formation
- Lung biopsy — fungal hyphae invading the lung parenchyma

Therapy
- Intravenous amphotericin. After a test i.v. dose of 1 mg, an infusion of 0.25 mg/kg/day is started, increasing to 1.0 mg/kg/day — total dose 2–4 g. The alternatives, miconazole 600 mg i.v. 8-hourly, or ketoconazole 200 mg 12-hourly orally, are less potent
- Oxygen
- Natamycin inhalation 2.5 mg in 1 ml saline 6-hourly
- Prognosis is very poor

5.18 Pulmonary eosinophilia

A group of conditions characterized by:
- fluffy, transient wedge-shaped or reticulonodular shadows on chest X-ray
- blood eosinophilia
- sputum eosinophilia is frequent

5.18   Pulmonary eosinophilia

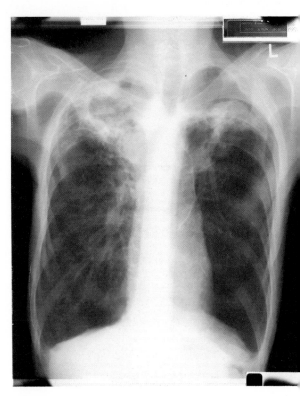

Fig. 147 *(a) Large aspergilloma in an old tuberculous cavity the left apex. Note the crescent of air outlining the upper margin of the intracavity fungal ball.*

These conditions can be divided into those that present with and those that present without asthma.

With asthma

- Allergic aspergillosis — (60%) patients have a simultaneou type I and type III immune response
- A cause is rarely found in the other 40%

5.18 Pulmonary eosinophilia

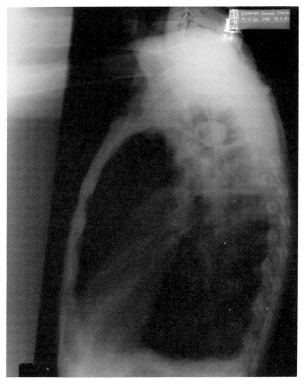

Fig. 147 *(b) Lateral view of aspergilloma.*

Without asthma

These patients can be divided into 3 diagnostic groups:
* simple pulmonary eosinophilia
* tropical eosinophilia
* polyarteritis nodosum

1 Simple pulmonary eosinophilia (Loeffler's syndrome)
This is a short illness with chest X-ray changes. Causes include fungi, worms and drugs.

5.18 Pulmonary eosinophilia

Fungi. This illness may be caused by:
- aspergillus

Worms. These may be of the following types:
- *Ascaris lumbricoides*
- *Ancyclostoma*
- *Taenia saginata*
- *Trichuris*
- *Toxocara canis*

Drugs causing simple pulmonary eosinophilia may be:
- sulphonamides
- nitrofurantoin
- antituberculous therapy (PAS)
- gold
- penicillin
- aspirin

2 Tropical eosinophilia
Signs include cough, dyspnoea, fever, chest pain; the main cause is filariasis in the tropics. Symptoms include very high IgE levels and a high eosinophil count. Tropical eosinophilia responds to diethylcarbamazine 1 mg/kg/day, rising to 6 mg/kg/day after 3 days. Treatment should continue for 3 weeks.

3 Polyarteritis nodosum (PAN)
Pulmonary eosinophilia occurs with or without asthma. Other features of PAN (hypertension, neuropathy, nephritis) are usually present (see **5.19**).

5.19 Musculoskeletal diseases and the lung

Rheumatoid arthritis

Pulmonary complications of rheumatoid arthritis include:
- pleurisy and pleural effusion — relatively common, may be recurrent, usually small. Low glucose in pleural fluid
- obliterative bronchiolitis
- bronchiectasis
- fibrosing alveolitis

5.0 Some important diseases

5.19 Musculoskeletal diseases and the lung

- rheumatoid nodules — may be multiple, can cavitate, may disappear
- Caplan's syndrome — coal worker's pneumoconiosis with large nodules (2–3 cm) which may cavitate

Systemic lupus erythematosus (SLE)

Respiratory complications of this rare disease are:
- pleurisy and effusion. These are both common, the effusions being usually small, often bilateral
- lupus pneumonia — bilateral patchy pneumonia with fever, tachypnoea and hypoxia
- restrictive ventilatory defect. The small lung volumes and breathlessness are due to respiratory muscle weakness. Lung fibrosis is rare, but bilateral basal atelectasis is common

Therapy for any of the pulmonary complications is with steroids — prednisone 60 mg daily initially, reducing to 10–15 mg per day as a maintenance dose. Alternate-day therapy may be possible.

Polyarteritis nodosum (PAN)

Pulmonary features may include:
- asthma
- eosinophilia
- pneumonic episodes

These occur in addition to some of the other features of the disease:
- hypertension
- nephritis (haematuria and proteinuria)
- mononeuritis multiplex
- rheumatoid-like arthropathy

Steroids are used to treat PAN — initially prednisolone 60 mg daily reducing to a maintenance dose of 10–15 mg daily. Prognosis depends upon renal involvement.

5.0 Some important diseases

5.19 Musculoskeletal diseases and the lung

Ankylosing spondylitis

Pulmonary complications include:
- restriction of chest wall movement due to fusion of costovertebral joints — $\downarrow$FEV$_1$, $\downarrow$FVC $\uparrow$FEV$_1$/FVC%, $\downarrow$TLC
- apical fibrosis which may cavitate, simulating tuberculosis
- aspergilloma may grow in these apical cavities
- pneumonia is often the terminal event due to restricted chest wall movements
- respiratory failure particularly after abdominal surgery when respiration, which is almost entirely diaphragmatic, becomes 'splinted' due to pain thus causing hypoventilation

Systemic sclerosis

Pulmonary complications are often seen late in the disease:
- pulmonary fibrosis
- aspiration pneumonia if the oesophagus is affected

Therapy of systemic sclerosis is ineffective although steroids are usually tried for the pulmonary fibrosis. Physiotherapy and antibiotics are needed for aspiration.

Kyphoscoliosis

Causes
- Congenital abnormality with or without vertebral abnormalities
- Thoracoplasty (Fig. 148)
- Idiopathic (Fig. 149)
- Neuromuscular and skeletal diseases — tuberculosis, ankylosing spondylitis, osteoporosis, osteomalacia, polio

Clinical features
Scoliosis causes more respiratory problems than kyphosis. Severe scoliosis can lead to:
- progressive dyspnoea (reduced FVC and TLC increases the work of breathing)
- hypoxia due to ventilation/perfusion mismatch and alveolar hypoventilation
- pulmonary hypertension leading to cor pulmonale
- respiratory failure — usually in fifth or sixth decades

5.19   Musculoskeletal diseases and the lung

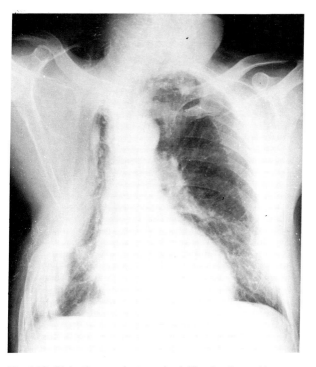

Fig. 148 *Right thoracoplasty and calcification from old tuberculosis.*

Therapy
- Surgical correction will improve lung function in the young
- Antibiotics for secondary infection
- Diuretics for cor pulmonale
- Oxygen — for acute problems, long-term domiciliary therapy may also help

Prognosis
Unfortunately, the long-term prognosis of severe scoliosis is often poor once cardio-respiratory complications appear.

5.20   Cystic fibrosis

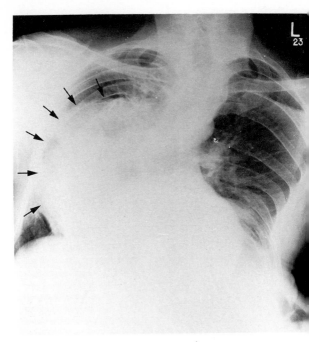

Fig. 149 *Severe kyphoscoliosis — vertebrae arrowed.*

5.20   Cystic fibrosis (mucoviscidosis, fibrocystic disease)

This recessive hereditary disease affects the mucus and non-mucus secreting exocrine glands. Most of the clinical features relate to the increased viscosity of mucus. The biochemical abnormality is unknown. The homozygote state occurs in approximately 1:2000 live births; 1:25 of the population are heterozygous for the recessive gene, making this condition one of the more common hereditary abnormalities. At present, there is no reliable way of identifying the heterozygote. However, parents of an affected child must both be heterozygotes, thus they have a 1:4 risk of any further children being affected.

5.0 Some important diseases

5.20 Cystic fibrosis

Clinical features (Fig. 150)

The disease nearly always presents with some of the following features, affecting both children and adults.

Children
- Recurrent upper and lower respiratory infections leading to bronchiectasis typified by cough with purulent sputum,

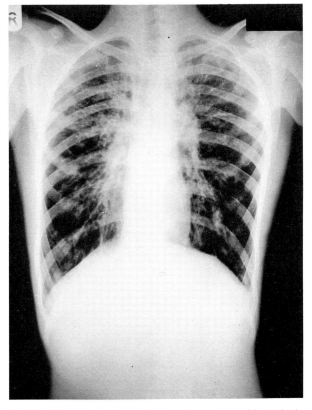

Fig. 150 *Fibrocystic disease, hyperinflated lungs with marked upper-zone interstitial shadowing and basal tramline shadows due to bronchiectasis.*

wheeze, progressive dyspnoea, haemoptysis and finger clubbing
- Intestinal obstruction (meconium ileus) in neonates, recurrent abdominal pain in older children
- Faecal impaction and rectal prolapse
- Malabsorption and growth retardation due to pancreatic insufficiency
- Hepatic cirrhosis
- Nasal polypi

Adults
- Recurrent bronchiectatic infection
- Pneumothorax
- Respiratory failure and cor pulmonale
- Sinusitis
- Pancreatic insufficiency
- Impotence

Investigations

Chest X-ray
A chest X-ray shows hyperinflation with scattered areas of infection and gradual destruction of lung architecture.

Sweat sodium and chloride
Measured after stimulation with pilocarpine, sweat sodium and chloride values for each of over 70 mEq/l are diagnostic in children but less reliable in adults. For this reason a fludrocortisone suppression test is preferred in adults. Give 0.1 mg daily; if sweat sodium does not fall the diagnosis is made.

Faecal fat excretion
Fat excretion is increased with pancreatic disease.

Therapy (for adults)

Out-patient
- Regular postural drainage
- Bronchodilators if there is a reversible element to the airways obstruction
- Antibiotics according to sensitivity of organism
- Oral pancreatic enzyme replacement for malabsorption

5.0 Some important diseases

5.20 Cystic fibrosis

- High-protein, high-calorie diet, low fat intake
- Extra fat-soluble vitamins (A, D, E, K)
- Extra salt in hot weather

In-patient
In-patient therapy is required primarily for acute infections, but also sometimes for pneumothoraces. The main organisms are likely to be *Pseudomonas aeruginosa, Staphylococcus aureus* and *Haemophilus influenzae*. Prolonged intravenous antibiotics are given. Until the results of sputum and blood culture are available, the following should be given:

- i.v. flucloxacillin 500 mg 6-hourly, and tobramycin (3–5 mg/kg/day) together with either carbenicillin 5 mg 6-hourly or azlocillin 5 mg 6-hourly
- antibiotics have also been given successfully by nebulization-carbenicillin 1 g 12-hourly and gentamicin 80 mg 12-hourly
- physiotherapy with postural drainage
- oxygen (humidified) 35%
- salbutamol nebulization
- diuretics (if there is cor pulmonale)

Prognosis

With vigorous physiotherapy and antibiotic therapy the prognosis for children has greatly improved, with 25% living into their third, and a few into their fourth decade.

5.21 Goodpasture's syndrome

The circulating IgG anti-glomerular basement membrane antibodies responsible for the glomerulonephritis cross-react with the alveolar basement membrane.

Clinical features

- Haemoptysis ⎫
- Hypoxia ⎬ Due to intrapulmonary haemorrhage
- Diffuse pulmonary infiltrates ⎭
- Renal failure due to glomerulonephritis

5.0 Some important diseases

5.21 Goodpastures' syndrome

Therapy

Early treatment is essential from among the following:
- prednisolone 60 mg daily
- cyclophosphamide 3 mg/kg/day
- azathioprine 1 mg/kg/day
- repeated plasma exchange

This is highly specialized therapy and should only be undertaken in specialist units.

6.0 Other clinical problems

6.0 Other clinical problems

6.1 Giving up smoking

There are about eighteen million smokers in the UK. The prevalence is gradually falling; of males 52% were smokers in 1972 and 45% in 1978. Only 25% of professional or managerial staff now smoke, whereas over 50% of manual workers still do so.

Risks of smoking

Tobacco smoking is directly implicated in the aetiology of the three commonest causes of premature death in males in western countries:

- coronary thrombosis
- chronic bronchitis
- lung cancer

It is also implicated as a cause of numerous other diseases, including:

- cerebrovascular disease
- peripheral vascular disease
- peptic ulceration
- carcinoma of tongue, nasopharynx, larynx, oesophagus, bladder and pancreas

Overall it is estimated that smoking causes over 50 000 deaths and the loss of 50 million working days annually in the UK. The cost to the National Health Service of treating smoking-related diseases is estimated at £155 million a year (1981 figures). 40% of smokers die before reaching retirement compared with only 15% of non-smokers.

Reasons for smoking

Social pressure of peer groups at school or at work is the usual reason for starting to smoke. Once started, the reason for continuing is nicotine addiction. This addiction and the physical discomfort associated with withdrawal make giving up difficult. The two other principle harmful ingredients in cigarettes are tar (a mixture of thousands of compounds) and carbon monoxide.

6.0   Other clinical problems

6.1   Giving up smoking

Reducing the incidence of smoking-related diseases

There are 2 main ways this can be done. The first is to accept
smoking as inevitable, but to make it safer. The patient should
be encouraged to switch to one of the following:
- filter tips, which now make up 90% of cigarettes sold. They
  produce less tar, but the carbon monoxide yield is variable
- low tar (< 10 mg) cigarettes. Tar yields are published by the
  government agencies (they range from 3–28 mg/cigarette)
- cigars or a pipe. These have a higher tar yield, but most pipe
  or cigar smokers are 'non-inhalers'

Problems with this approach are:
- smokers who switch to cigars often continue to inhale and
  may not, therefore, reduce their risks
- smokers who switch to lower tar cigarettes tend to increase
  inhalation
- lower tar content does not reduce the harmful effects of
  carbon monoxide
- lower tar may reduce lung cancer, but probably does not
  reduce bronchitis and emphysema

Experiments with tobacco substitutes have been dropped
because of poor market response.

The second way to reduce the incidence of smoking-related
disease is to try and reduce the number of smokers by actively
discouraging the young from starting and by helping adults to
give up.

Most people who have given up smoking have done so through
their own will-power. Numerous other methods are available to
help smokers give up but it must be emphasized that none
stand any chance of being successful unless the patient really
wants to stop. Most therapies have short-term success rates of
30–80%, but the long-term results of all show about a 20%
one year success rate. Effectiveness is as follows:
- group therapy and smokers clinics — long-term results
  consistent at 15–20%
- hypnosis ⎫
- MD6 filters ⎭ effectiveness unproven
- nicotine chewing gum — this is claimed to have a success
  rate of 70% during therapy but 25% at one year. It is

6.1 Giving up smoking

available on private prescription. Results are only available from a few centres, thus further evaluation is necessary.
• behavioural therapy. The success rates of both electrical aversion and rapid smoking are unproven.

There is no doubt that the doctor is most likely to persuade the patient to give up smoking when the patient has developed symptoms such as haemoptysis, chest pain or shortness of breath, or when a member of his family develops a smoking-related disease such as lung cancer. Unfortunately, all too often one sees a patient with lung cancer who stopped smoking either a 'few months ago' or 'last week'.

Checking whether patients still smoke

It is essential to be able to check by carboxyhaemoglobin (COHb) estimation whether the patient has given up smoking or not. It is unreliable to believe what the patient says. Two methods of testing this are available, by:
• direct blood measurement — this is time consuming
• breath measurement (Ecolyser) — this gives an immediate read out.

The 2 methods correlate well, the Ecolyser being ideal for out-patients. All town dwellers have measurable COHb levels but those of smokers are much greater.

6.2 Respiratory failure

Types

Respiratory failure is defined as an arterial oxygen tension of less than 60 mmHg (8 kPa) with a normal or low Pa_{CO_2} (Type I) or with an elevated Pa_{CO_2} (> 50 mmHg 6.7 kPa; Type II).

Causes

Type I
Hypoxia with normal Pa_{CO_2} due primarily to ventilation/perfusion mismatch. This can be caused by:
• asthma (in the early stage of an attack)

6.2   Respiratory failure

- pneumonia
- left ventricular failure
- 'pure' emphysema
- fibrosing alveolitis
- adult respiratory distress syndrome

Type II
Hypoxia with elevated Pa_{CO_2} due primarily to hypoventilation with or without associated ventilation/perfusion mismatch. Causes are:
- chronic obstructive bronchitis
- asthma (in a very severe attack)
- drugs depressing respiratory drive, e.g. opiates or barbiturates
- neurological conditions, e.g. myasthenia gravis, Guillain-Barré syndrome, cervical cord lesions, or polio
- chest injuries, e.g. flail chest

Clinical features
The clinical features are those of the underlying disease together with the symptoms and signs of hypoxia alone (Type I) or hypoxia and hypercapnia superimposed (Type II)

Symptoms and signs of hypoxia
- Tachycardia
- Cyanosis
- Confusion leading to coma

Symptoms and signs of hypercapnia
- Headaches
- Tachycardia
- Warm, vasodilated peripheries
- Flapping tremor
- Confusion and coma
- Papilloedema
- Peripheral oedema

Investigations

The following investigations are particularly important in evaluating and treating patients with suspected respiratory failure:
- arterial blood gases and pH (note inspired O_2 content)

6.0 Other clinical problems

6.2 Respiratory failure

- lung function tests — peak flow rate, FEV_1, FVC and gas transfer
- sputum examination and culture
- chest X-ray

Therapy

Oxygen therapy (see also **7.4**)

In normal man, including those with Type I respiratory failure, respiratory drive is stimulated mainly by hypercapnia and, to a lesser extent, by hypoxia. In patients with chronic hypercapnia (mainly chronic bronchitics) and many with Type II respiratory failure, the hypercapnic drive has been 'poisoned', thus hypoxia is the main respiratory driving force. Since correction of hypoxaemia in these patients may remove the ventilatory drive, the main aim of therapy must be to correct hypoxaemia without causing hypoventilation and thus aggravating respiratory failure. However, it should be emphasized that *alleviation of hypoxia is essential*. This is achieved by closely monitoring the $Paco_2$. The $Paco_2$ gives an excellent guide to ventilation because it depends almost entirely on alveolar ventilation whereas the Pao_2 depends mainly upon ventilation/perfusion matching and, to a lesser extent, alveolar ventilation.

Controlled oxygen therapy in respiratory failure. The routine is as follows.

1. Take sample for blood gases while the patient is breathing air. If the $Paco_2$ is normal or low (Type I), 35% (or more) oxygen therapy can be given. Careful control of oxygen therapy is not going to be necessary. If the $Paco_2$ is elevated (Type II), 24% oxygen is given. In this case, oxygen therapy will have to be carefully watched.
2. Recheck blood gases after 20 minutes of breathing oxygen. If the $Paco_2$ has risen significantly (> 5 mmHg) on 24% oxygen and the patient is still hypoxic, it may be necessary either to introduce a respiratory stimulant such as doxapram or, rarely, to institute artificial ventilation. If the $Paco_2$ is lower or steady, oxygen can be increased to 28%.
3. Recheck blood gases after 20 minutes of breathing 28% oxygen. If the $Paco_2$ has remained constant or fallen, increase to 35% oxygen. If the $Paco_2$ has risen > 5 mmHg, return to 24% oxygen.

4. After 20 minutes, recheck the $Pa\text{CO}_2$ whilst breathing 35% oxygen. If the $Pa\text{CO}_2$ has risen, return to 28% oxygen and recheck blood gases 20 minutes later.
5. If, using this regimen it is not possible to correct hypoxaemia without the $Pa\text{CO}_2$ rising, i.e. the hypoventilation is worsening, then doxapram (0.5–4.0 mg/min using a 2 mg/ml in 5% dextrose solution i.v.) should be given to stimulate respiration. If this fails, then the patient will need to be paralysed, intubated and ventilated artificially. Before this is done, one must consider a large number of factors including the potential reversibility of the underlying condition and the quality of the patient's life over the last few months.

If blood gas analysis is not available, then the rebreathing technique for $Pa\text{CO}_2$ estimation can be used to monitor therapy. Failing this, the level of consciousness and general ventilatory effort should be used. A patient who is in respiratory failure should be constantly stimulated to keep him awake. **All sedatives are absolutely contraindicated**.

Antibiotics
The likeliest infecting organisms are *H. influenzae* or the *Pneumococcus*. Therefore ampicillin 500 mg 6-hourly, or cotrimoxazole 960 mg 12-hourly, or oxytetracycline 500 mg 6-hourly, are the antibiotics of choice, unless, on the result of Gram stain and culture of sputum, there are grounds to suspect other organisms. If the infection was acquired in hospital, antibiotics must be given for *Staphylococci* (flucloxacillin) and Gram-negative organisms (gentamicin or tobramycin).

Physiotherapy
Physiotherapy is given to aid sputum production, clear airways and rouse the patient. Percussion to the chest 4-hourly is usually sufficient. Tracheal suction can be performed with a soft catheter. Fibreoptic bronchoscopy is used for 'bronchial toilet' if the first two are inadequate.

Bronchodilators
Aminophylline 5 mg/kg i.v. is given over 20 minutes, then 0.5 mg/kg/h continuously **and** nebulized salbutamol 5 mg or terbutaline 5 mg or fenoterol 2.5 mg 4-hourly.

6.0 Other clinical problems

6.2 Respiratory failure

Steroids (hydrocortisone) are often given i.v. but there is little evidence to support their use other than in asthma.

Treat other complications
- Right ventricular failure — frusemide 80 mg i.v. stat. — then a regular oral dose
- Atrial fibrillation — digoxin 0.25 mg 12-hourly orally initially, then reduce dose according to renal function
- Pneumothorax — intercostal tube with underwater seal

Respiratory stimulants

Possible indications for use of respiratory stimulants are:
- Drug overdose — opiates, barbiturates, benzodiazepines
- Respiratory failure secondary to chronic obstructive airways disease
- Neuromuscular disorders — myasthenia gravis, poliomyelitis

Types. Adults suspected of drug overdose with opiates should be treated with naloxone 0.4 mg–1.2 mg i.m. Myasthenia gravis should be treated with anti-cholinesterases such as neostigmine or pyridostigmine. Severe hypoventilation due to other drugs or neuromuscular disorders requires artificial ventilation. When a respiratory stimulant is wanted because of other causes of alveolar hypoventilation such as chronic bronchitis, the drug of choice is doxapram, given as a continuous infusion of 0.2–0.4 mg/min of the 2 mg/ml solution in 5% dextrose. The most notable possible side-effects are convulsions, which are dose-related. A new encouraging drug is almitrine. Nikethamide and vanilic acid are now rarely, if ever, used.

If respiratory stimulants fail, artificial ventilation is needed, either until the drug causing hypoventilation has worn off, or until the infection and bronchospasm precipitating the respiratory failure have been controlled.

6.3 Adult respiratory distress syndrome ('shock lung')

This term is often applied to patients in whom there is non-cardiogenic pulmonary oedema caused by increased pulmonary capillary permeability. There are numerous factors which may cause this increased permeability.

6.0 Other clinical problems

6.3 Adult respiratory distress syndrome

Causes

- Aspiration of gastric acid (Mendelsohn's syndrome)
- Inhalation of smoke and fumes
- Virus pneumonia
- Gram-negative sepsis
- Cardiopulmonary bypass
- Re-expansion oedema after a pneumothorax
- Heroin overdose
- Near-drowning
- Hypothermia
- Altitude sickness
- 'Neurogenic' after head injuries
- Major trauma
- Acute pancreatitis

Clinical features

- Very ill patient
- Tachycardia
- Tachypnoea
- Hypoxia in spite of high-concentration oxygen therapy
- Bilateral alveolar shadowing on chest X-ray with characteristic sparing of the costophrenic angles, the heart size is normal (Fig. 151)
- Type I respiratory failure
- Need for artificial ventilation in order to provide adequate oxygenation
- Pulmonary artery wedge pressure (measured by a Swan-Ganz catheter) is normal

Therapy

- Oxygenation and artificial ventilation are the mainstays of therapy, sometimes with the addition of positive end expiratory pressure (PEEP). Great care should be taken not to overhydrate the patient and hence make the pulmonary oedema worse
- Circulatory support with inotropes such as dopamine or dobutamine if necessary
- High-dose steroids are often given, but there is little proof that they alter the outcome (50% mortality)

6.0 Other clinical problems

6.3 Adult respiratory distress syndrome

- Treatment of the underlying disease
- Aggressive treatment of intercurrent infection

6.4 Cardiac failure

The respiratory physician is frequently confronted with the problem of cardiac failure. This may be either pulmonary oedema due to left ventricular failure presenting as breathlessness (Fig. 152), or right ventricular failure secondary either to left ventricular failure (congestive cardiac failure) or

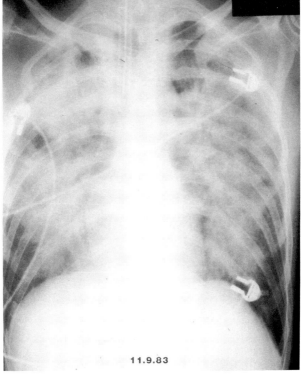

Fig. 151 *Non-cardiogenic pulmonary oedema in a patient with the adult respiratory distress syndrome.*

6.4 Cardiac failure

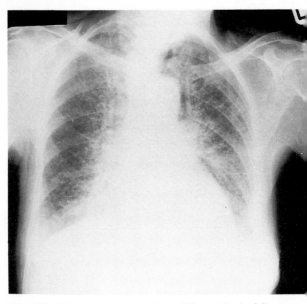

Fig. 152 *Pulmonary oedema due to left ventricular failure.
Note cardiomegaly, bilateral pleural effusions, hilar flare and
interstitial shadowing.*

secondary to pulmonary hypertension caused by chronic lung
disease (cor pulmonale).

Causes

Left ventricular failure
- Ischaemic heart disease
- Cardiomyopathy
- Valvular heart disease
- Hypertension
- Renal failure
- Overhydration
- Thyrotoxicosis

Cor pulmonale
- Chronic bronchitis and emphysema

6.0 Other clinical problems

6.4 Cardiac failure

- Recurrent pulmonary embolism
- Any chronic lung disease resulting in pulmonary hypertension

Clinical features

Left ventricular failure
- Tachycardia
- Gallop rhythm
- Large heart
- Basal crepitations
- Pulmonary oedema on chest X-ray

Congestive cardiac failure
- Raised JVP ⎫
- Large liver ⎬ in addition to signs above
- Peripheral oedema ⎭

Cor pulmonale
- Symptoms and signs of chronic pulmonary disease
- Large right ventricle
- Loud pulmonary second heart sound
- Raised JVP
- Large liver
- Peripheral oedema
- No signs of left ventricular failure

Therapy

- Identify and treat underlying cause
- Bed rest
- 35% oxygen (unless in Type II respiratory failure)
- Frusemide 80 mg i.v. initially, then orally to control oedema
- Digoxin only to control atrial fibrillation if present
- Vasodilator therapy if the above measures fail

6.5 Sleep apnoea

Types (Fig. 153)

Sleep apnoea is defined as the occurrence of 12 apnoeic episodes of at least 10 seconds duration per hour. The apnoeic episodes occur during rapid eye movement (REM) sleep. Sleep apnoea occurs 10 times more frequently in men than women.

6.0 Other clinical problems

6.5 Sleep apnoea

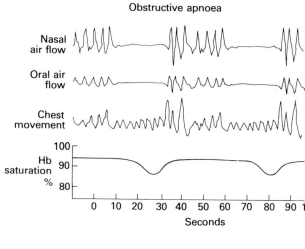

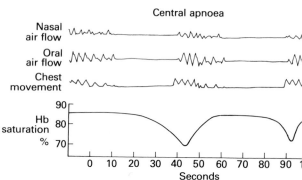

Fig. 153 *Sleep apnoea. In obstructive apnoea note that although there is continuous chest wall movement due to airways obstruction, usually in the nasopharynx, there is no airflow in or out of either the nose or the mouth, hence the arterial oxygen content falls. In central apnoea the CNS drive to breath is temporarily interrupted hence chest wall movement also stops.*

6.0 Other clinical problems

6.5 Sleep apnoea

Two main types are recognized (both may be seen in the same patient).

Central apnoea
There is neither chest wall movement nor airflow at the nose or mouth. This implies defective respiratory drive within the CNS. It is most often seen in young babies, particularly the premature. It is one of the possible aetiologies of 'cot death'.

Obstructive apnoea
There is no airflow at the nose or mouth, but normal or increased chest wall movement. This implies upper airways obstruction occurring in the oro- or naso-pharynx.

Causes of obstructive sleep apnoea

* Obesity
* Acromegaly
* Myxoedema
* Superior vena caval obstruction
* Large tonsils and adenoids
* Idiopathic — the largest group

Clinical features of obstructive sleep apnoea

* Snoring
* Drowsiness in the day
* Morning headache — due to hypoxia and hypercapnia
* Intellectual deterioration
* Personality changes
* Mental problems and impotence
* Enuresis
* Abnormal movements during sleep and sleep walking
* Cardiac dysrhythmias, rarely leading to sudden death
* Polycythaemia
* Pulmonary hypertension and cor pulmonale
* Often found in 'blue bloaters' — the 'Pickwickian syndrome'
* May masquerade as narcolepsy

Investigations

* Observe sleep

6.0 Other clinical problems

6.5 Sleep apnoea

- Place a tape recorder in the bedroom to record patterns of breathing
- Continuously monitor oxygen saturation with an ear oximeter or T_cPo_2 transcutaneous Po_2 electrode
- Use nasal and oral thermisters to record whether there is airflow at nose or mouth
- Record chest wall movement
- Record the EEG continuously

Therapy

The following are some of the treatments which have been tried; their number reflects their lack of effectiveness:
- treatment of any associated disease
- weight loss
- medroxyprogesterone — CNS stimulant and fat redistribution
- protriptyline — decreases amount of REM sleep
- intubation of oronasopharynx
- pharyngeal wall surgery
- tonsillectomy and removal of adenoids if these are responsible for obstruction
- tracheostomy
- use of apnoea alarms for babies with central apnoea to alert their parents so that they can waken the child

6.6 Thermal injury (smoke inhalation)

Most deaths in fires are caused by suffocation. However, anyone who has been exposed to toxic fumes and smoke should be observed for at least 24 hours in hospital in case they develop complications.

Clinical features

Acute airways obstruction
The patient wheezes and coughs up blackened sputum. This reaction is due to mucosal oedema and bronchospasm.

Pulmonary oedema
The patient is acutely short of breath without wheezing. This reaction is often delayed up to 24 hours after exposure.

6.0 Other clinical problems

6.6 Thermal injury (smoking inhalation)

Therapy

Treatment is rarely necessary for the acute airways obstruction apart from physiotherapy and a bronchodilator once the patient has been removed from the source of smoke. The following treatment is required if pulmonary oedema develops:

• remove from source of smoke
• oxygen (humidified) 35% oxygen
• i.v. hydrocortisone 200 mg
• take care not to overhydrate
• artificial ventilation may be necessary
• antibiotics for superadded infection

6.7 Paraquat poisoning

Clinical features

The mortality from an oral overdose of the weedkiller, paraquat, is around 50% when taken either in error, or as a suicide attempt. Initially, there is burning of the mouth, lips and an oesophagitis; over the next few days pulmonary oedema, haemorrhage and fibrosis with hyaline membrane formation occur. Hypoxaemia and death usually follow despite artificial ventilation. Jaundice and renal failure also occur. Great care must be taken in the use and storage of this substance; its commercial names and strengths in the UK are:

• Gramoxone (20%)
• Dextrone (20%)
• Weedol (2.5%)

Therapy

(a) Reduce absorption
  • gastric and whole gut lavage
  • give large amounts of Fuller's earth orally (or Bentonite)
(b) Aid clearance
  • forced diuresis
  • haemodialysis or charcoal haemoperfusion
(c) Give oxygen — adequate to maintain Pao_2 — too much may enhance toxicity.

The degree of therapeutic intervention depends upon the blood paraquat level.

6.8   Opportunistic pneumonia and pyrexia in the immunosuppressed

Causes

Immunosuppressed patients, such as those with lymphoma undergoing chemotherapy, those who have undergone renal or other transplantation, frequently develop chest infections. Often the infection is acquired in hospital, Gram-negative bacteria of the *Klebsiella, Enterobacter, Seratia* group are frequent. *Escherichia, Pseudomonas* and *Proteus* are commonl* found. Patients with acute myeloblastic leukaemia or myeloma also tend to have infections with Gram-positive bacteria such as *Staph. aureus, Strep. pneumoniae* or Group D *Streptococcus*. Tuberculosis must always be kept in mind.

In addition to these organisms which may cause infection in patients with normal host defences there are numerous organisms, in particular *Pneumocystis carinii*, which do not infect normal lungs, but which infect the lungs of the immunosuppressed:

- bacteria — *Nocardia*
- fungi   — *Candida*
             Aspergillus
             Cryptococcus
- viruses   — *Cytomegalovirus*
             Herpes simplex
             Varicella zoster
- Protozoa — *Pneumocystis carinii*
             Toxoplasma gondii

Clinical features

Although there may be **no** obvious clinical features other than fever, the common features are:

- fever
- cough — usually unproductive
- increasing dyspnoea
- hypoxia — leading to Type I respiratory failure
- patchy consolidation on chest X-ray

6.0 Other clinical problems

6.8 Opportunistic pneumonia and pyrexia

Investigations

The following investigations to identify the site and cause of
infection are mandatory:
* chest X-ray
* sputum Gram stain and culture (bacterial and viral)
* sputum auramine or ZN stain
* nasal and throat swab culture (bacterial and viral)
* microscopy and culture of urine
* blood cultures
* swab of any infected site for culture
* blood for baseline serological and virological investigation
  which can be repeated after 10 days to see if there is any
  rising titre

Despite these investigations, an infecting organism is identified
in only about 30% of cases unless more aggressive techniques
such as transbronchial lung biopsy and bronchoalveolar lavage
are performed and in some cases, open lung biopsy is
necessary. Even then, the yield is increased to only 70%.

Therapy

In the absence of definite bacteriological guidance the following
regimen is used to provide a broad-spectrum cover, in particular
for Gram-negative organisms:
* tobramycin, a loading dose of 100 mg i.v. followed by a
  maintenance dose of 80 mg 8-hourly i.v.
* together with mezlocillin 5 g 6-hourly i.v., and
* cotrimoxazole 3.84 g 12-hourly (to cover pneumocystis)

The doses are adjusted according to blood levels and renal
function.

* If all cultures are unhelpful and the patient has not responded
  by day 3, add a third antibiotic, cefotaxime 1 g 6-hourly i.v.
  If these drugs have failed by day 6, replace them with the
  following combination:
* erythromycin 500 mg 6-hourly and
* metronidazole 400 mg 8-hourly

Failure to respond to these drugs indicates possible fungal or
tuberculous infection.

6.0 Other clinical problems

6.8 Opportunistic pneumonia and pyrexia

Anti-fungal therapy
The treatment of choice is amphotericin B which should be
given as a 1 mg test dose with pulse and temperature being
monitored for 4 hours. If there is no adverse reaction, an
intravenous infusion over 6 hours of 0.25 mg/kg body weight,
increasing to 1 mg/kg body weight is given, giving 500 ml of
mannitol before and after infusion to lessen renal damage. If
the patient is in renal failure, then miconazole 600 mg i.v.
6-hourly should be used rather than amphotericin.

Anti-tuberculous therapy
A specific (but not first line) anti-tuberculous regimen consists
of isoniazid, ethambutol and pyrazinamide. These drugs are
ineffective against other bacteria whereas rifampicin and
streptomycin are broad-spectrum antibiotics as well as
powerful anti-tuberculous drugs.

6.9 The acquired immunodeficiency syndrome (AIDS)

AIDS is caused by human T cell lymphotropic virus III (HTLV III)
invading and killing helper (T4) lymphocytes. After a long
period (length unknown) an unknown proportion of infected
people will develop AIDS. The main pulmonary complication
caused by the immunosuppression is pneumonic illness, usually
(85%) caused by *Pneumocystis carinii*, either alone (67%) or
together with other organisms. The other pulmonary
complication of AIDS is the development of Kaposi's sarcoma,
seen in 8% of cases.

Common pathogens in AIDS

Pneumocystis carinii (85%)
CMV (17%)
Mycobacterium avium intracellulare (17%)
Legionella pneumophila
Pyogenic bacteria — e.g. *Pneumococcus*,
   Staph. aureus
Mycobacterium TB   (<10%)
Herpes simplex virus
Fungi

6.0 Other clinical problems

6.9 The acquired immunodeficiency syndrome (AIDS)

Clinical features

These may include:
- persistent dry cough for 2–3 weeks
- fever
- malaise, often for several months
- increasing breathlessness
- often generalized lymphadenopathy
- progressive weight loss
- patient in high-risk group, e.g. homosexual or bisexual, haemophiliac, i.v. drug abuser
- oropharyngeal candidiasis
- hypoxia — at first only on exertion, later at rest — if untreated leading to type I respiratory failure
- bilateral crackles — however, these are not always found
- Kaposi's sarcoma in some patients

Investigation

- HTLV III antibody — this is a marker of HTLV III infection and is found in 97% of patients with AIDS, but also in about 30% of the homosexual population who do not currently suffer from AIDS.
- Chest X-ray — pneumocystis — bilateral diffuse ground glass alveolar or interstitial appearance is classical, but many patterns including a normal X-ray are possible. Focal segmental shadows suggest bacterial causes.
- Lung function tests — look for reduced gas transfer (TLCO, KCO).
- Blood gases — ↓ Pao_2 with normal or ↓ $Paco_2$.
- Sputum — Gram stain
  - culture and sensitivity
  - Ziehl-Neelsen or Auramine stain for AFB.
- Fibreoptic bronchoscopy for bronchoalveolar lavage and transbronchial lung biopsy, both of which should be examined specifically for pneumocystis with silver methenamine, and for CMV and Mycobacteria.

With these techniques, a causative agent can be found in 90% of cases of AIDS; in the others open lung biopsy is indicated — this is also required for a diagnosis of intrapulmonary Kaposi's sarcoma.

6.9   The acquired immunodeficiency syndrome (AIDS)

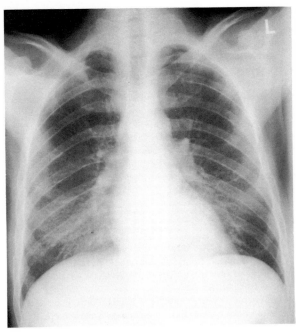

*Pneumocystis pneumonia in patient with AIDS — bilateral groun
glass appearance in both lower and mid-zones.*

Therapy

As yet there is no effective therapy for the underlying conditio
of AIDS, which is universally fatal. However, the prognosis fo
an individual episode of AIDS pneumonia is relatively good —
75% survival of first episode. The mean prognosis from the
first pneumonic episode to death is about 6 months. In additio
to oxygen the following therapies are indicated.
- *Pneumocystis carinii* — i.v. cotrimoxazole (20 mg
  Trimethoprim/kg/day) in divided doses for 3 weeks, or
  Pentamidine 4 mg/day (more toxic).
- Cytomegalovirus — Hyperimmune serum and DHPG are bot
  undergoing clinical trials.

6.0 Other clinical problems

6.9   The acquired immunodeficiency syndrome (AIDS)

- Herpes simplex — Acyclovir is successful in some early cases.
- Fungi — i.v. Amphotericin B.
- Mycobacterium avium intracellulare — conventional anti-TB regimens have little success. Clofazimine and Ansamycin are being evaluated.
- Conventional therapy is given for pyogenic bacterial or TB.
- There is no effective therapy for intrapulmonary Kaposi's sarcoma.

Prophylaxis against recurrent pneumocystis. Pneumocystis tends to recur, hence either cotrimoxazole 2 tabs 12 hourly, or fansidar 1 tablet weekly can be given.

Complications. Hypoxic respiratory failure (type I). The prognosis if artificial ventilation is required is extremely poor (15% survival of that episode).

Considerable time and patience is needed in counselling the patient, his relatives and allaying the anxiety of hospital staff.

Therapy

7.1   Cough therapy

Cough suppressants

There are over 100 compound preparations prescribed or purchasable over the chemist's counter for cough. They often contain a mixture of an expectorant, a cough suppressant, a sympathomimetic, a sedative and an antihistamine. The use of such mixtures is not recommended. Before a cough suppressant is prescribed, assess whether the accompanying risk of sputum retention is really desirable. Coughing is one of the most useful and effective lung drainage and defence mechanisms. It is particularly useful in bronchitis, pneumonia and bronchiectasis. Nevertheless, should a suppressant be needed (perhaps to enable a good night's sleep), codeine linctus 10 ml nocte or pholcodeine linctus 10 ml nocte should be tried. The main side-effect is constipation. In diabetes, prescribe the diabetic preparations which are diluted with chloroform water rather than syrup. Often a cough is due to smoking. It is, therefore, best to try and persuade the patient to give up the habit.

Opiates

Opiates are effective cough suppressants but they are also addictive and respiratory suppressants. In the UK they are controlled drugs and their prescription must meet with the requirements of the Misuse of Drugs regulation (1973). The main legal requirement for out-patient use is that the prescription must be written, signed and dated in the hand of the prescriber who must give his own name and address. The following must also be written:
1. name and address of patient;
2. the form and strength of the preparation;
3. the dose in words and figures;
4. the total quantity of the drug in both words and figures.

In the UK hospital ward these drugs are kept in a separate double-locked cupboard (Dangerous Drugs Act (DDA) cupboard). Each dose must be accounted for in a book signed by 2 people, one of whom must be a doctor or trained nurse.

Despite their side-effects, opiates are very useful for their

7.0 Therapy

7.1 Cough therapy

analgesic and cough-suppressant actions, especially in patients with malignant lung disease. The dose is titrated against the symptoms.

Preparations include:
- diamorphine linctus 3 mg/5 ml
- methadone linctus 2 mg/5 ml

NB Methadone **mixture** used in the treatment of drug addicts is 2½ times the strength of the linctus.

Expectorants

There is no evidence that any drug aids expectoration. However, drugs given for this purpose include ammonium chloride and ipecacuanha. The rationale of such use is that emesis caused by these compounds is accompanied by simultaneous mucus expectoration.

Mucolytics

There are numerous drugs available to help chronic bronchitics expectorate less viscid sputum by breaking down disulphur bonds. Numerous claims are made but it is doubtful whether any such compound is effective.

7.2 Bronchodilators

β-Adrenergic receptors

Most, if not all, cells have surface β-adrenergic receptors. There is debate as to whether the number of these are diminished in asthmatics as compared with normal people. It appears, however, that chronic β-agonist therapy reduces and steroid therapy increases the number of receptor sites.

The stimulation of β_1 receptors causes cardiac effects such as tachycardia, whereas the stimulation of β_2 receptors leads to bronchial smooth muscle relaxation and bronchodilation. The use of non-selective β agonists such as adrenaline and isoprenaline which have β_1 and β_2 effects has greatly diminished since the introduction of the selective β_2 drugs, which have less cardiac stimulant action.

Examples of β_2 stimulants are:
• salbutamol
• terbutaline
• fenoterol
• rimiterol
• reproterol

For efficacy there is little to choose between any of these. With the exception of rimiterol, they are effective for up to 5 hours and any claimed advantage of one over another is usually theoretical rather than of clinical relevance. Their action is longer lasting than that of isoprenaline because the side-chains attached to their basic molecule render them relatively resistant to enzymatic breakdown by cathechol-orthomethyl transferase (COMT). The preferred route of administration is by inhalation, either from a metered dose aerosol, or a dry powder device, or from a nebulizer. The metered dose aerosol containing a mixture of the drug and fluorinated hydrocarbons as propellant is the commonest mode employed (Fig. 154). After inhaling from the aerosol, the onset of action is rapid (within minutes) reaching a peak effect within ½–1 hour followed by a plateau effect lasting about 2 hours, which wears off after 4–5 hours when a further dose is given.

Tablet forms of some of these drugs are available but the total dose is higher, thus leading to more side-effects and the onset of action is delayed (½ hour). Their only advantage is in ensuring that patients who are unable to use an inhaler properly receive adequate therapy. However, this situation is now more unusual since dry-powder devices are available in addition to pressurized aerosols.

Side-effects
Side-effects of β_2 adrenergic drugs are dose related:
• fine muscular tremor
• feeling of nervousness
• tachycardia and occasionally cardiac dysrhythmias
• headache
• dizziness
• hypokalaemia

7.0 Therapy

7.2 Bronchodilators

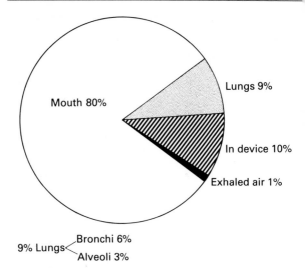

Fig. 154 *Deposition of drug after metered dose aerosol inhalation (after Newman S.P et al. 1981).*

Guidelines for β_2 adrenergic bronchodilator therapy
- Exclude thyrotoxicosis or severe ischaemic heart disease first
- Teach the patient how to use the metered dose inhaler
- Prescribe either salbutamol 200 μg
  or terbutaline 500 μg
  or fenoterol 360 μg
  (i.e. 2 puffs) 6-hourly for routine therapy

It is worth noting that side-effects such as tremor found with 1 drug do not necessarily occur if the patient is changed to another.

- For troublesome nocturnal asthma, slow-release preparations are available, salbutamol spandets 8 mg 12-hourly, or terbutaline slow-acting 7 mg 12-hourly. There is little evidence to support their use
- In acute asthma attacks give regular nebulizations of salbutamol 5 mg or terbutaline 5 mg or fenoterol 2.5 mg over 15 minutes, because in acute exacerbations not only is it difficult for the patient to inhale from a metered dose

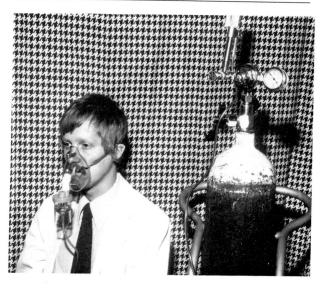

Fig. 155 *Nebulization via a Hudson mask.*

inhaler but also the drug penetration is less than by
nebulization (Fig. 155). The total dose given this way is
higher, and hence, side-effects are much more common
For patients who have difficulty in using the metered dose
inhalers, use fenoterol or salbutamol dry-powder devices or a
terbutaline spacer. However, as these are expensive, some
time should be spent observing and instructing the patient in
the use of the metered dose inhaler first.

Anticholinergics

Ipratropium bromide
Ipratropium is an anticholinergic agent with bronchodilator
properties, yet has no apparent effect on the cardiovascular
system in therapeutic doses. It is effective both in most
asthmatics and some patients with chronic obstructive airways
disease. As the onset of action is slow (1 hour peak) this agent
may not be as popular with patients as β agonists, because it
does not give immediate relief to their symptoms. There is a
little evidence that the effects of ipratropium and β agonists are

additive. Ipratropium may be administered either by metered dose inhaler (40 μg 6-hourly) or via nebulizer (0.1–0.5 mg 6-hourly). No adverse effect on sputum viscosity or on mucociliary clearance have been reported.

Contraindications
- Atropine hypersensitivity

Precautions
- Glaucoma
- Prostatic hypertrophy

Side-effects
- Dry mouth
- Urinary retention
- Constipation
- Bronchospasm (in a very few)

Overdose
- Tachycardia
- Palpitations

Aminophylline

Intravenous aminophylline is the drug of choice in severe, acute asthma attacks. There is currently a resurgence of interest in oral aminophylline, particularly the longer-acting formulations. Aminophylline causes bronchial smooth muscle relaxation by increasing levels of intracellular cyclic AMP, possibly through its action as a phosphodiesterase inhibitor. There are 2 main problems with aminophylline therapy. First, absorption and breakdown is very variable. Second, the toxic range is only a little above the therapeutic range. Ideally, therefore, therapy should be monitored with regular blood theophylline levels.

The main indication for slow-release aminophylline is when trying to improve severe morning 'dips' when they are probably the best preparation currently available.

Side-effects
The side-effects of aminophylline are:
- nausea and vomiting (most common)

- tachycardia and cardiac dysrhythmias
- convulsions

Precautions
Aminophylline should be given with caution in patients with liver disease, or those who are epileptic, or lactating. It is worth noting that there is a small group of patients (mainly photographic workers) who are allergic to ethylene diamine, one of the components of aminophylline. In such cases aminophylline causes a rash and makes bronchospasm worse — i.v. lysine theophylline or oral theophylline therapy may provide an answer.

Dose

Acute asthma. 250–500 mg (5 mg/kg) slowly i.v. over 10–15 minutes followed, if necessary, by a slow continuous infusion of 500 μg/kg/h.

Maintenance. Slow-release oral tablets 225–450 mg 12-hourly dose being monitored by blood levels.

7.3 Anti-allergic drugs

Sodium cromoglycate

The mode of action of sodium cromoglycate is also uncertain. One theory is that it prevents mediator release (histamine, prostaglandin and leukotrienes) from mast cells after an antigen challenge. It is a useful drug in most atopic (extrinsic) asthmatics and also in a few intrinsic asthmatics. It should also be tried in patients with exercise-induced asthma. Sodium cromoglycate is not useful during an asthma attack, only for preventing them. There are few, if any, notable side-effects. The recommended dose is 20–40 mg 6-hourly, given as spincaps in a spinhaler. There is a metered dose inhaler (2 mg 6-hourly) which is more convenient for patients to use.

Ketotifen

This drug's mode of action is claimed to be similar to that of sodium cromoglycate. It is given by mouth and may need up to

7.3 Anti-allergic drugs

4 weeks before its full benefit is achieved. Its efficacy in adult
is generally disappointing. Because it also has the properties c
an antihistamine, its main side-effects are:
- dry mouth
- sedation

Ketotifen should be taken with care if combined with alcohol,
or if the patient is going to drive. The recommended dose is
1 mg 12-hourly which can be doubled if necessary.

Corticosteroids

How these drugs cause bronchodilation is unknown; one theo
is that they cause 'up regulation' of the number of β adrenerg
receptors, another is that by blocking arachidonic acid
production, they stop production of mediators such as
prostaglandins and leukotrienes. They are very effective
bronchodilators. Their onset of action is slow (12–24 hours).

Steroids block the late response to inhaled allergens, but do n
affect the immediate response, nevertheless they lessen the
likelihood of further attacks. The aim is to control asthma with
as low a dose of steroids as possible — preferably given only
via a metered dose inhaler without any oral therapy. However
a few patients require tablet therapy.

Dose
Inhaled beclomethasone dipropionate 100 μg 6-hourly, or
betamethasone 200 μg 6-hourly. In severe asthmatics, inhale
beclomethasone 500 μg 6–12 hourly.

Only with inadequate control, i.v. hydrocortisone 200 mg, or
oral prednisone in doses adequate to control symptoms, initia
40 mg daily.

Precautions
- Diabetes mellitus
- Hypertension
- Tuberculosis (active or inactive)

Side-effects of oral steroids
- Increased appetite and weight gain
- Osteoporosis and vertebral collapse

7.0 Therapy

7.3 Anti-allergic drugs

- Hypertension
- Diabetes mellitus
- Cataracts
- Increased risk of infection
- Myopathy
- Adrenal suppression

The main side-effect to occur with inhaled steroids is an increased prevalence of oral candidiasis. This is more common with high-dose steroid inhalers (Becloforte = beclomethasone 500 μg; with this dose there is also some adrenal suppression).

7.4 Oxygen therapy

The ultimate cause of death in respiratory disease is almost always tissue hypoxia. When assessing the need for oxygen therapy or the response to oxygen, it is important to remember that it is the oxygen content and saturation of blood that is more important than the absolute value of the oxygen tension (Pa_{O_2}). Tissue oxygen delivery is determined by the arterial oxygen content and the cardiac output.

Factors adversely affecting oxygen delivery

Decreased cardiac output
- Cardiogenic shock and left ventricular failure
- Hypovolaemic shock

Reduced arterial oxygen content
- V/Q abnormalities in the lung — hypoxia is often completely reversed by increasing the oxygenation of the relatively poorly ventilated parts of the lung
- Alveolar hypoventilation — oxygen may overcome the hypoxia but the hypercapnia will remain, and in certain situations it may be worsened, e.g. 'blue bloaters'.
- Anaemia
- Smoking (high COHb)
- Factors affecting haemoglobin dissociation (pH and Pa_{CO_2})

Abnormal local distribution
- Vasodilation or vasoconstriction of local blood vessels

7.4 Oxygen therapy

Oxygen delivery methods

Ventimask (24%, 28%, 35%)
These masks work on the venturi principle (Fig. 156).
Depending on the flow rate of oxygen supplied to the mask,
24%, 28% or 35% oxygen is delivered to the patient. It is
necessary to give controlled oxygen therapy to chronic
bronchitics in respiratory failure because their hypercapnic
respiratory drive is limited (see **6.2**).

Pneumask, MC Mask, Nasal spectacles (40–60%)
All 3 of these methods deliver high concentration of oxygen
and are suitable for patients with conditions such as asthma,

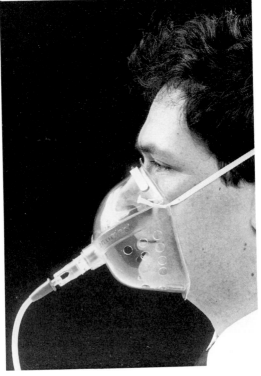

Fig. 156 *Venturi oxygen mask.*

pulmonary embolism, interstitial lung diseases and left
ventricular failure where the respiratory drive is normal.

Artificial ventilation
This is the only way in which extremely high (> 60%) oxygen
concentrations (with its risks of toxicity) can be delivered to
adults. Oxygen tents are used to give high concentrations to
children.

Side-effects and cautions

Hypercapnic respiratory failure (see **6.2**)
Patients with chronic bronchitis who hypoventilate rely only
upon hypoxic rather than hypercapnic respiratory drive. If this
hypoxic drive is abolished the hypoventilation may worsen,
leading to carbon dioxide narcosis and death.

Fire and explosion risk
Naked flames and smoking must be forbidden.

Oxygen toxicity
With high inspired oxygen concentration (> 50%) for 48–72
hours at least, there may be pulmonary capillary proliferation,
haemorrhage and hyaline membrane formation. This does not
occur with mask delivery as it is impossible to achieve high
enough oxygen delivery.

Rebound hypoventilation after stopping oxygen
Oxygen therapy is essential in the hypoxic patient. Once it has
commenced, it is important to give it continuously because
intermittent therapy may lead to 'rebound' hypoxia.

Retrolental fibroplasia (blindness)
This results from high oxygen concentrations given to
neonates.

7.5   Artificial ventilation

Aims

• Relief of hypoxia
• Control of hypercapnia

7.0 Therapy

7.5 Artificial ventilation

- Reducing the work of breathing
- Control of the airway and ease of removing secretions

Indications

Respiratory failure in a patient with potentially reversible lung disease. The decision to start artificial ventilation is taken on the basis of clinical deterioration with worsening hypoxia $\pm$ hypercapnia:
- increasing tachypnoea
- confusion
- hypotension
- physical exhaustion
- worsening cyanosis
- deteriorating blood gases — $\downarrow Pa_{O_2} \pm \uparrow Pa_{CO_2}$

Methods

Artificial ventilation should be undertaken by experienced physicians or anaesthetists in an Intensive Care Unit. Two main types of ventilators are used:
- volume cycled — a set volume is delivered each breath
- pressure cycled — a variable volume is delivered until a set pressure is reached

The shortcoming of the pressure-cycled machines is that they provide inadequate ventilation if there is airways obstruction or with poorly compliant lungs or if the endotracheal tube becomes kinked. Therefore, a volume-cycled ventilator is preferable. The minute volume of the humidified gas mixture is normally set at 6–9 litres at a rate of 15 breaths/minute. For 3–4 days ventilation is performed through a low-pressure, cuffed endotracheal tube, after this a tracheostomy should be considered if prolonged artificial ventilation is likely.

7.6 Antibiotics (Fig. 157)

Anti-bacterial drugs act in six main ways as detailed below. The first four are bactericidal, the last two groups are largely bacteriostatic.

7.6 Antibiotics

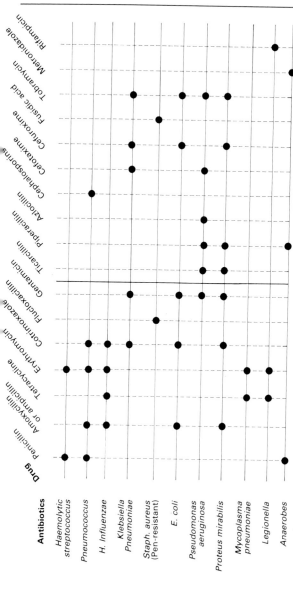

Fig. 157 Suggested usage of antibiotics based upon usual bacterial sensitivities and price. It should be noted that a choice from the first seven antibiotics, alone or in combination, covers almost all respiratory infections.

7.0 Therapy

7.6 Antibiotics

Interference with the bacterial cell wall
Penicillin and cephalosporins

Disruption of cell membrane
Nystatin, amphotericin

Interference with RNA polymerase
Rifampicin

Degradation of DNA
Metronidazole

Interference with folate manufacture
Sulphonamides and trimethoprim

Interference with protein synthesis on the ribosomes
Streptomycin, gentamicin (both bactericidal) erythromycin,
tetracycline, chloramphenicol, clindomycin (all bacteristatic)

Penicillins

The penicillins are bactericidal because they interfere with cell
wall synthesis.

Side-effects of all penicillins
- Diarrhoea
- Skin rashes
- Encephalopathy
- Sodium and water retention — with high doses
- Allergy — anaphylaxis

Penicillinase-sensitive penicillins
- Benzylpenicillin (Pen G): 300–600 mg 6-hourly i.m. or i.v.
- Phenoxymethylpenicillin (Pen V): 250–500 mg 6-hourly
  orally

Penicillinase-resistant penicillins
Most hospital-acquired staphylococci are penicillinase
producers and hence resistant to the 2 penicillins above. Thus,
use either:
- Flucloxacillin 250–500 mg 6-hourly p.o./i.m. or i.v., or
- Methicillin 1 g 6-hourly i.m. or i.v.

7.0 Therapy

7.6 Antibiotics

Broad-spectrum penicillins
These have Gram-positive and Gram-negative activity.
- Ampicillin 500 mg 6-hourly p.o. or i.v.
- Amoxycillin — better absorbed than ampicillin — 500 mg 8-hourly
- Piperacillin — good anti-pseudomonas activity — 200 mg/kg daily slowly i.v. or i.m.

Anti-pseudomonal penicillins
- Carbenicillin 5 g 4 to 6-hourly i.v.
- Ticarcillin 5 g 6-hourly i.v.
- Azlocillin 2 g 8-hourly i.v.

Cephalosporins

These broad-spectrum antibiotics are usually reserved for patients who are penicillin sensitive although 10% of them will also be sensitive to cephalosporins. Most of these drugs are inactive by mouth
- Cefuroxime 750 mg 8-hourly i.v. or i.m.
- Cefotaxime 1 g 12-hourly i.v. or i.m.

Side-effects are similar to those of the penicillins.

Tetracyclines

These broad-spectrum antibiotics are now used mainly in the therapy of acute on chronic bronchitis, mycoplasma, rickettsial or chlamydial infection.

Side-effects
- Deposition in growing teeth and bone causing yellow discolouration
- Renal failure
- Gastrointestinal upset

Do not give them to pregnant women, to children aged under 14 years or to patients with renal disease.

Aminoglycosides

Aminoglycosides are bactericidal antibiotics particularly useful against Gram-negative organisms.

7.0 Therapy

7.6 Antibiotics

- Gentamicin 2–5 mg/kg daily in divided doses 8-hourly i.m. or i.v.
- Tobramicin 3–5 mg/kg daily in divided doses 8-hourly i.m. or i.v.
- Amikacin 7.5 mg/kg 12-hourly i.m. or i.v.

Doses must be carefully regulated by blood levels. Gentamicin peak (1 hour) levels should not exceed 10 μg/ml with trough levels less than 2 μg/ml.

Side-effects
- Oto-vestibular toxicity
- Renal failure

Avoid use in pregnancy and myasthenia gravis. Use with care with diuretics which may be ototoxic.

Macrolides

Oral erythromycin 500 mg 6-hourly is used in penicillin-sensitive individuals. It is also the drug of choice in:
- whooping cough
- mycoplasma pneumonia
- psittacosis
- Legionnaire's disease

Side-effects
- Gastrointestinal upset
- Cholestatic jaundice

Sulphonamides and trimethoprim

Cotrimoxazole is a mixture of 5 parts sulphamethoxazole and 1 part trimethoprim.

It is active against *H. influenzae*, hence it is useful in chronic bronchitis. Dose — 960 mg 12-hourly, 3.84 g 12-hourly are used for pneumocystis infection.

Side-effects
- Gastrointestinal upset
- Skin rashes

- Bone marrow suppression
- Megaloblastic anaemia

Contraindications
- Pregnancy
- Renal or hepatic failure
- Blood diseases

Oral trimethoprim 200 mg 12-hourly is less toxic than cotrimoxazole but is effective in acute exacerbations of chronic bronchitis.

Metronidazole

Metronidazole is particularly useful against anaerobes, which may occur within a lung abscess or empyema.

Side-effects
- Gastrointestinal upset
- Antabuse effect with alcohol
- Leucopenia
- Peripheral neuropathy
- Dizziness and ataxia

Dose 400 mg 8-hourly orally or 500 mg 8-hourly i.v.

7.7   Anti-viral agents

There are few effective anti-viral agents, thus it is fortunate that most viral infections are self-limiting.

Idoxuridine

Idoxuridine is used for local application to the rash of herpes simplex or varicella zoster (shingles) but it must be applied early in the disease. It is too toxic for systemic use.

Vidarabine

Vidarabine is effective against chicken pox and shingles which may cause pneumonia in the immunosuppressed. Side-effects include gastrointestinal disturbance, ataxia, confusion and bone marrow suppression. It should not be used in pregnancy.

Dose 10 mg/kg daily for at least 5 days given by slow i.v. injection.

Acyclovir

Acyclovir is particularly useful for the therapy of herpes simplex pneumonia (or encephalitis). Side-effects include renal and liver failure and bone marrow suppression. The patient must be well hydrated and the dose reduced if there is renal impairment.

Dose 5 mg/kg over 1 hour, repeated every 8 hours.

7.8 Diuretics

The most commonly used diuretics are the 'loop' diuretics which inhibit resorption from the ascending loop of Henle.

Frusemide

For acute left ventricular failure, start with 40 mg i.v. (in cardiac failure there is gastric oedema and hence poor oral absorption). Potassium replacement therapy is often not required (unless K^+ is less than 3.5 mmol/l) except if the patient is receiving digoxin or has had a recent myocardial infarction. Normal dose orally is 20–80 mg once or twice daily but not after 4.00 pm so that the diuresis is over by bedtime.

Side-effects
- Potassium depletion — important in patients receiving digoxin or after a myocardial infarction
- Precipitation of liver failure in patients with cirrhosis
- Aggravation of gout
- Aggravation of diabetes mellitus
- May precipitate retention of urine if there is an enlarged prostate
- Deafness (with very large doses of the drug)
- Rashes
- Nephrotoxicity with simultaneous cephalosporin therapy

7.8 Diuretics

Bumetanide

This has a similar action to frusemide, but has the main advantages of being cheaper and having a shorter duration of action (useful for patients who go out a lot). Dose range orally is 0.5–2.0 mg once or twice daily.

Side-effect
These are the same as those for frusemide with the addition of myalgia if bumetanide is given in large doses.

Amiloride

A weak diuretic on its own, amiloride is often used with a thiazide or 'loop' diuretic to conserve potassium. Dose is 5–20 mg daily.

Cautions or contraindications
* Cirrhosis
* Diabetes
* Hyperkalaemia
* Renal failure

Side-effects
* Rashes
* Confusion

Spironolactone

Useful in situations where there is hyperaldosteronism, such as the following:
* cirrhosis
* nephrotic syndrome
* Conn's syndrome

It is also useful in refractory cardiac failure, when used together with 'loop' diuretics. Potassium supplements may lead to dangerous hyperkalaemia. The dosage is 100–200 mg daily initially.

Contraindications
* Hyperkalaemia
* Renal failure

7.0 Therapy

7.8 Diuretics

Side-effects
- Gastrointestinal disturbances
- Gynaecomastia

7.9 Digoxin

The cardiac glycosides are now almost entirely reserved for the control of atrial fibrillation. The commonest causes of atrial fibrillation are:
- ischaemic heart disease
- mitral valve disease
- thyrotoxicosis
- pulmonary embolism

The onset of atrial fibrillation may be associated with discomfort and shortness of breath due to cardiac failure. The loss of the atrial 'boost' reduces the cardiac output by 20% at an even ventricular rate. However, the ventricular rate at the onset of atrial fibrillation may be very rapid (180 beats/min), failing to permit adequate ventricular filling, hence the cardiac output may drop even more than 20%.

When very rapid control of atrial fibrillation is required, DC cardioversion is indicated. If this is not the case, try digoxin 0.75 mg i.v. over 30 minutes followed by 0.25 mg daily thereafter (less in the elderly). If gradual digitalization is needed, 0.25 mg 12-hourly for 3 days with 0.25 mg daily thereafter is usually sufficient. Give lower doses in the elderly and those with renal disease.

Precautions
Use digoxin with caution in the following:
- elderly — monitor blood levels: toxic levels are more than 2.5 nmol/l; sample taken at least 6, and preferably 8, hours after dose
- renal failure — monitor blood levels
- hypokalaemia
- recent myocardial infarction
- hypothyroidism
- hypercalcaemia

The daily dose of digoxin should be omitted if the patient's pulse is less than 60 beats/min.

Side-effects
- Nausea and appetite loss
- Vomiting
- Dysrhythmias and heart block

7.10 Respiratory side-effects of therapy

Asthma

If certain groups of drugs are administered to asthmatics, it must be done with great caution because they may precipitate acute attacks.

β-blockers ('Non-selective')
- Propranolol
- Oxprenolol
- Timolol
- Nadolol
- Sotalol
- Prenalterol

Asthma is less commonly worsened by the 'selective' β-blockers.
- Atenolol
- Acetabutolol
- Metoprolol
- Practalol

Analgesics
- Aspirin
- Indomethacin
- Phenylbutazone
- Morphine
- Pentazocine
- Diamorphine

Dyes
- Tartrazine

Muscle relaxants
- Suxamethonium
- Tubocurare
- Pancuronium

7.0 Therapy

7.10 Respiratory side-effects of therapy

Fibrosing alveolitis

Local radiotherapy (Fig. 158)

Cytotoxic agents
- Methotrexate
- Busulphan
- Bleomycin
- Melphalan
- Cyclophosphamide
- BCNU

Anti-microbials
- Nitrofurantoin (is also a rare cause of acute pulmonary oedema)
- Sulphasalazine

Hypotensive agents
- Hexamethonium
- Practalol
- Oxprenolol

Anti-rheumatic agent
- Gold

Anti-arrhythmic drugs
- Amiodarone
- Tocainide

If lung changes occur due to any of these drugs, the drug should immediately be stopped and steroid therapy (prednisone 40 mg/d) started. With all these drugs, patients should have regular chest X-rays and lung function tests, to watch for infiltrates and changes in the gas transfer (TLCO).

Pulmonary embolism

Oral contraceptives
High-dose oestrogen pills (over 50 μg) are associated with an increased risk of pulmonary embolism. In this country, oral contraceptives now contain a maximum of 50 μg ethinyloestradiol in combination with a progestogen. Alternatively, progestogen-only oral contraceptives are

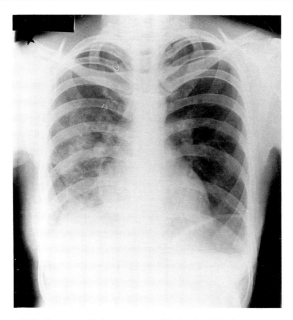

Fig. 158 *Acute radiation pneumonitis in the right lung following radiotherapy for a carcinoma in the right breast.*

prescribed. This reduction in oestrogen appears to have lessened the risk of pulmonary embolism. However, they should not be prescribed for any woman with a history of pulmonary embolism and should be discontinued immediately if one occurs. Alternative methods of contraception should then be advised.

Stilboestrol and tamoxifen
Patients given these drugs to treat prostatic or breast carcinoma are at an increased risk of pulmonary embolism.

Adult respiratory distress syndrome (ARDS)

Oxygen
The breathing of a high concentration of oxygen (> 50%) for prolonged periods (> 24 hours) can lead to the adult

7.11 Drug interactions.

Drug	Toxic action with	Potentiated by	Action blocked by	Potentiates	Blocks
Chloramphenicol			Barbiturates	Phenytoin Anticoagulants	
Corticosteroids	Ethacrynic acid Live vaccines		Barbiturates Phenytoin Rifampicin		
Cyclophosphamide				Neuromuscular blockers	
Digoxin	Allopurinol		Rifampicin Aminoglycosides Antacids		
Frusemide			Indomethacin Phenytoin	Methyldopa Guanethidine Clonidine	
Isoniazid			Antacids	Phenytoin Alcohol	
Methotrexate		Probenecid Salicylates			
Metronidazole	Alcohol	β blockers		Anticoagulants Clonidine Ethacrynic acid Frusemide	
Methyldopa		Clonidine		Sympathomimetics — both direct and indirect NB cough mixtures	

Drug					
Penicillins / Phenylbutazone			Probenecid / Tetracyclines / Barbiturates	Alcohol / Anticoagulants / Hypoglycaemic agents / Phenytoin	Guanethidine / Thiazides
Phenytoin / Rifampicin		Chloramphenicol	Anticoagulants	Anticoagulants	Oral contraceptives / Anticoagulants / Oral contraceptives / Corticosteroids
Salicylates			Probenecid	Anticoagulants / Hypoglycaemic agents / Methotrexate	Digoxin / Probenecid
Sulphonamide				Hypoglycaemic agents / Phenytoin	
Sympathomimetics direct and indirect	Tricyclic antidepressants / Guanethidine / Methyldopa / Mono-amine oxidase inhibitors				Guanethidine

respiratory distress syndrome (ARDS). Initially there is cough, then dyspnoea; reduction in vital capacity and pulmonary infiltration follow. *V/Q* mismatch occurs with increasing hypoxaemia. Care must, therefore, be taken when giving oxygen, particularly to neonates and patients on ventilators.

Lupus-like syndrome

Features are arthralgia, skin rash, pleurisy with effusion and pulmonary infiltration; positive ANF.

Hypotensive agents
• Hydralazine

Anti-arrhythmic agent
• Procainamide

Intrapulmonary haemorrhage

Penicillamine rarely causes nephritis and intrapulmonary haemorrhage — similar to Goodpasture's syndrome.

Appendices

Appendices

1   NHS prescriptions (UK only)

1   NHS prescriptions (UK only)

The present cost of each item on a prescription is £2.00. Many patients with respiratory diseases such as asthma need frequent multiple prescriptions, so it is cheaper for them to buy a 'season ticket' (Prepayment Certificate) costing £11.00 for 4 months or £30.50 for a year. To buy a season ticket a patient needs form EP95 (EC 95 in Scotland), obtainable from a Post Office, local Social Security office, chemist or from the local Family Practitioner Committee office.

Free prescriptions are available to the following:
• pensioners
• children under 16 years old and students over 16 years old still at school or college
• pregnant women
• mothers with children under 1 year old
• those receiving family income supplement or supplementary benefit
• war or service pensioners needing prescriptions for their accepted disablement

They are also available to those suffering from the following conditions:
• permanent fistulae (including caecostomy, colostomy or ileostomy)
• conditions requiring replacement therapy, e.g. Addison's disease or other forms of hypoadrenalism — diabetes mellitus; hypoparathyroidism; myasthenia gravis; myxoedema
• epilepsy
• a continuous physical disability which prevents the patient leaving home without the help of another person (temporary disabilities do not count)

Many patients with chronic lung disease, such as adult asthmatics do not qualify for free drugs, although they need continuous therapy. They should, therefore, be advised to buy season tickets.

2   Benefits available in the UK

About 60 different cash benefits are available in the UK, some of which may help patients in times of need. Some of those benefits to which those with respiratory diseases may be entitled are given below, together with the relevant DHSS booklet reference. Booklets are available from either local DHSS offices or from the DHSS Leaflet Unit, PO Box 21, Stanmore, Middlesex HA7 1AY.

- Family income supplement-FIS 1
- Supplementary benefit — SH1
- Sickness benefit — N1 16
- Invalidity benefit — N1 16A
- Non-contributory invalidity pension (NCIP) N1 210 (men and single women) or N1 214 (married women)
- Hospital patients travelling expenses — H11
- Leaflet N1 9 explains how many benefits are reduced by a stay in hospital
- Industrial disablement benefit — claims form B1 100A (accident), B1 100B (prescribed disease), B1 100(Pn) (pneumoconiosis or byssinosis). Information in leaflets N1 6 (disablement), N1 2 (industrial diseases), N1 3 (pneumoconiosis and byssinosis)
- Industrial death benefit N1 10 contains information. Claim is made by special form given by the Registrar of Deaths or on form B1 200 obtainable from a social security office
- Workmen's compensation supplement (Pre 1948) WS1
- Pneumoconiosis, byssinosis and miscellaneous disease benefits (Pre 1948) PN1
- Attendance Allowance — N1 205
- Invalid Care Allowance — N1 212
- Mobility Allowance — N1 211
- Assistance with fares to work — DPL 13

Medical evidence for social security purposes (sickness certificates)

In the UK, doctors are required to give the following certificates free of charge under the National Health Service Acts. The forms are available from Family Practitioner Committees or Health Boards.

2 Benefits available in the UK

Form Med 3 (Doctor's statement)
The usual form filled in after examination of patients by GPs or doctors in out-patients (whichever has the overall clinical responsibility). The length of certified sickness may last from days up to 6 months initially.

Form Med 5 (Doctor's special statement)
Form Med 5 is given when Med 3 is inappropriate, e.g. to give a certificate for a past period of illness or where the GP has not examined the patient but is relying upon a recent report from another doctor.

For both forms Med 3 and Med 5 the diagnosis must be stated as precisely as possible, unless the doctor considers it inadvisable on medical grounds to disclose the true diagnosis to the patient. In that case, the diagnosis may be stated less precisely, but a separate form, Med 6 (notice to Divisional Medical Officer), should be completed concurrently with the statement concerned.

If a doctor would like a second opinion, form RM7 (Doctor's request to Divisional Medical Officer) should be completed. This is unnecessary for civil servants or postal workers who are subject to their own special procedures.

Form Med 10
This is used only for in-patients. It can be signed by a doctor, dentist or any other member of the hospital staff who has been authorized to do so. A certificate is provided as soon as possible after admission. On discharge a certificate is issued when the patient is unfit for work and he is either referred back to his GP or will be seen in the out-patients department within a week. If the patient is unfit and is not being seen for more than a week, form Med 3 is required. Similarly, if the patient is fit for work on discharge, or is expected to be fit within 2 weeks, form Med 3 and not Med 10 should be given to the patient on discharge.

3 Foreign travel

All patients with chronic respiratory diseases should take out private insurance before they travel abroad. This should include cover for pre-existing diseases, which will be at a higher premium but is still worthwhile. Residents of the UK should obtain DHSS leaflet SA 30 *Medical treatment during visits abroad*. This gives information about obtaining form E111 for free treatment, or treatment at reduced cost, in other EEC countries.

4   Notification of infectious diseases

In the UK, the following diseases are notifiable by law to the local medical officer responsible for environmental health, using the statutory form and the telephone where appropriate:

- anthrax
- cholera
- diptheria
- dysentery
- encephalitis (acute)
- food poisoning (or suspected)
- infective jaundice
- Lassa fever
- leprosy
- leptospirosis
- malaria
- Marburg Virus Disease
- meningitis (acute)
- ophthalmia neonatorum
- paratyphoid
- plague
- poliomyelitis
- rabies
- relapsing fever
- scarlet fever
- smallpox
- tetanus
- tuberculosis
- typhoid
- typhus
- viral haemorrhagic fever (Ebola)
- whooping cough
- yellow fever

Although many of these diseases may have respiratory symptoms, tuberculosis is that most commonly diagnosed by the respiratory physician. All forms of the disease are notifiable, including those patients (or contacts) who are treated on the basis of a strongly positive tuberculin test in the absence of overt disease (chemoprophylaxis).

5   Useful addresses

The following are some useful addresses in the UK. The blank pages at the end of the book are for readers to insert other addresses.

ASH (Action on Smoking and Health)
5–11 Mortimer Street
London W1N 7RH
Tel: 01-637 9843

The Asthma Society and Friends of the Asthma Research
   Council
12 Pembridge Square
London W2 4EH
Tel: 01-229 1149 or 01-221 2347

Asthma Research Council
12 Pembridge Square
London W2 4EH
Tel: 01-229 1149 or 01-221 2347

British Thoracic Society
30 Britten Street
London SW3 6NN
Tel: 01-352 2194

Cardiothoracic Institute
Brompton
London SW3
Tel: 01-352 8067

Chest, Heart and Stroke Association
Tavistock House North
Tavistock Square
London WC1
Tel: 01-387 3012

Health Education Council
78 New Oxford Street
London WC1
Tel: 01-637 1881

Appendices

5 Useful addresses

Pneumoconiosis Medical Panel
194 Euston Road
London NW1
Tel: 01-387 2858

Poisons centres

LONDON: New Cross Hospital
             Avonley Road
             London SE14
             Tel: 01-639 4380

EDINBURGH: The Royal Infirmary
             Edinburgh 3
             Tel: 031-229 2477

CARDIFF: The Cardiff Royal Infirmary
             Cardiff CF2 1SZ
             Tel: 0222-492233

BELFAST: The Royal Victoria Hospital
             Belfast
             Tel: 0232-40503

DUBLIN: Jervis Street Hospital
             Dublin 1
             Tel: 01-748782

6   Further reading

Bienenstock J. (1984) *Immunology of the Lung and Upper Respiratory Tract*. McGraw Hill, New York.

Clark T.J.H. (Ed.) (1981) *Clinical Investigation of Respiratory Diseases*. Chapman and Hall, London.

Cotes J.E. (1979) *Lung Function*, 4th edition. Blackwell Scientific Publications, Oxford.

Crofton J. & Douglas A. (1981) *Respiratory Diseases*, 3rd edition. Blackwell Scientific Publications, Oxford.

Emerson P. (Ed.) (1981) *Thoracic Medicine*. Butterworths, London.

Forgacs P. (1978) *Lung Sounds*. Baillière Tindall, London.

Hughes D. & Empey D. (1981) *Lung Function for Clinicians*. Academic Press, London.

James G. & Studdy P. (1981) *Colour Atlas of Lung Disease*. Wolfe Medical, London.

Saunders K.B. (1977) *Clinical Physiology of the Lung*. Blackwell Scientific Publications, Oxford.

Scadding J.G. & Mitchell D.N. (1985) *Sarcoidosis*, 2nd edition. Chapman and Hall, London.

Stradling P. (1981) *Diagnostic Bronchoscopy*, 4th edition. Churchill Livingstone, London.

Sykes M.K., McNicol M.W. & Campbell E.J.M. (1976) *Respiratory Failure.* Blackwell Scientific Publications, Oxford.

West J.B. (1981) *Pulmonary Pathophysiology — The Essentials*, 2nd edition. Williams & Wilkins, Baltimore.

Index

Note: Page numbers in *italics* refer to figures and/or tables.

Index

Index

Index

Index

354

Index

Index

Index

Index

Index

Index

Index

Index